ABC of
Clinical Haematology

Third Edition

13

ABCseries

The revised and updated ABC series – written by specialists for non-specialists

- With over 40 titles, this extensive series provides a quick and dependable reference on a broad range of topics in all the major specialities

- An easy-to-use resource, covering the symptoms, investigations, treatment and management of conditions presenting in your day-to-day practice

- Full colour photographs and illustrations aid diagnosis and patient understanding of a condition

- Each book in the new series now offers links to further information and articles, and a new dedicated website provides even more support

- A highly illustrated, informative and practical source of knowledge for GPs, GP registrars, junior doctors, doctors in training and those in primary care

For further information on the entire ABC series, please visit:

www.abcbookseries.com

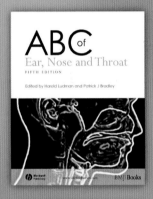

ABC of Ear, Nose and Throat
FIFTH EDITION
Edited by Harold Ludman and Patrick J Bradley

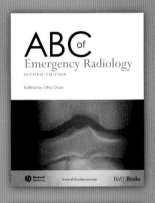

ABC of Emergency Radiology
SECOND EDITION
Edited by Otto Chan

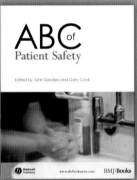

ABC of Patient Safety
Edited by John Sandars and Gary Cook

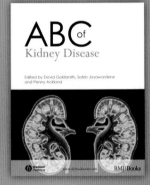

ABC of Kidney Disease
Edited by David Goldsmith, Satish Jayawardene and Penny Ackland

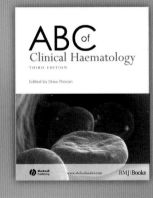

ABC of Clinical Haematology
THIRD EDITION
Edited by Drew Provan

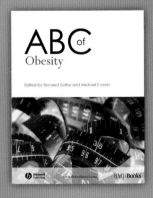

ABC of Obesity
Edited by Naveed Sattar and Michael E Lean

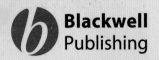

Blackwell Publishing

BMJ | Books

ABC of
Clinical
Haematology

Third edition

EDITED BY

Drew Provan
Senior Lecturer in Haematology
Barts and The London School of Medicine
London, UK

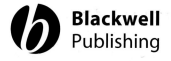 **Blackwell** Publishing

BMJ|Books

© 2007 by Blackwell Publishing Ltd
BMJ Books is an imprint of the BMJ Publishing Group Limited, used under licence

Blackwell Publishing, Inc., 350 Main Street, Malden, Massachusetts 02148-5020, USA
Blackwell Publishing Ltd, 9600 Garsington Road, Oxford OX4 2DQ, UK
Blackwell Publishing Asia Pty Ltd, 550 Swanston Street, Carlton, Victoria 3053, Australia

The right of the Author to be identified as the Author of this Work has been asserted in
accordance with the Copyright, Designs and Patents Act 1988.

First published 1998
Second edition 2003
Third edition 2007

1 2007

Library of Congress Cataloging-in-Publication Data
ABC of clinical haematology / edited by Drew Provan. -- 3rd ed.
    p. ; cm.
  Includes bibliographical references and index.
  ISBN 978-1-4051-5353-9
  1. Hematology--Outlines, syllabi, etc. I. Provan, Andrew.
  [DNLM: 1. Hematologic Diseases--diagnosis. 2. Hematologic Diseases--
physiopathology. 3. Hematologic Diseases--therapy. WH 120 A134 2007]

  RC633.A23 2007
  616.1'5--dc22

                                              2006035608

ISBN: 978-1-4051-5353-9

A catalogue record for this title is available from the British Library

Cover image of human red blood cells in a vein is courtesy of iStockphoto.com

Set in 9.25/12 pt Minion by Sparks, Oxford – www.sparks.co.uk
Printed and bound in Singapore by Markono Print Media, Pte Ltd

Associate Editor: Vicki Donald
Editorial Assistant: Victoria Pittman
Production Controller: Rachel Edwards

For further information on Blackwell Publishing, visit our website:
www.blackwellpublishing.com

The publisher's policy is to use permanent paper from mills that operate a sustainable
forestry policy, and which has been manufactured from pulp processed using acid-free and
elementary chlorine-free practices. Furthermore, the publisher ensures that the text paper
and cover board used have met acceptable environmental accreditation standards.

Contents

Contributors

Belinda Austen

Specialist Registrar in Haematology, University Hospital Birmingham NHS Foundation Trust, Birmingham, UK

Paul A Cahalin

Specialist Registrar in Haematology, Manchester Royal Infirmary, Manchester, UK

Fiona Clark

Consultant Haemato-Oncologist, Queen Elizabeth Hospital, Birmingham, UK

Mark Cook

Consultant Haemato-Oncologist, Queen Elizabeth Hospital, Birmingham, UK

Charles Craddock

Professor of Haemato-Oncology, Queen Elizabeth Hospital, Birmingham, UK

Tyrell G J R Evans

Senior Lecturer, King's College School of Medicine and Dentistry, London, UK

Adele K Fielding

Senior Lecturer/Honorary Consultant in Haematology, Royal Free and University College Medical School, London, UK

John M Goldman

Fogarty Scholar, Haematology Branch, National Institutes of Health, Bethesda, MD, USA

Anthony R Green

Professor of Haemato-Oncology, Cambridge Institute for Medical Research, Cambridge, UK

Andrew P Haynes

Senior Lecturer in Haematology, Nottingham University Hospitals Trust, Nottingham, UK

A Victor Hoffbrand

Emeritus Professor of Haematology, Royal Free and University College Medical School, London, UK

David M Keeling

Consultant Haematologist, The Churchill Hospital, Oxford, UK

Carolina Lahoz

Specialist Registrar, Barts and The London, Queen Mary's School of Medicine and Dentistry, London, UK

R J Leisner

Consultant Haematologist, Great Ormond Street Hospital for Children NHS Trust and University College London Hospitals NHS Trust, London, UK

Samuel J Machin

Professor of Haematology, Haemostasis Research Unit, University College London, London, UK

Jim Murray

Consultant Haematologist and Honorary Senior Lecturer, University Hospital Birmingham NHS Foundation Trust, Birmingham, UK

Adrian C Newland

Professor of Haematology, Barts and The London, Queen Mary's School of Medicine and Dentistry, London, UK

Simon O'Connor

Consultant Haematopathologist, Nottingham University Hospitals Trust, Nottingham, UK

Bella R Patel

Clinical Research Fellow, Royal Free and University College Medical School, London, UK

Drew Provan

Senior Lecturer in Haematology, Barts and The London, Queen Mary's School of Medicine and Dentistry, London, UK

Marie A Scully

Lecturer in Haematology, Haemostasis Research Unit, University College London, London, UK

Bronwen Shaw

Specialist Registrar in Haematology, Nottingham University Hospitals Trust, Nottingham, UK

Charles R J Singer

Consultant Haematologist, Royal United Hospital, Bath, UK

George S Vassiliou

Specialist Registrar in Haematology, Ipswich Hospital, Ipswich, UK

Sir David J Weatherall

Regius Professor of Medicine Emeritus, Weatherall Institute of Molecular Medicine, University of Oxford, Oxford, UK

John A Liu Yin

Professor in Haematology, Manchester Royal Infirmary, Manchester, UK

Preface to Third Edition

In the three years since the second edition of the *ABC of Clinical Haematology*, there have been further advances in our understanding and therapies for many haematological diseases. For some disorders new classification systems have been devised. For many disorders molecular techniques have provided major diagnostic tools and greater insight into the pathogenesis of the diseases themselves.

However, despite the complexity of modern clinical haematology, the aim of the *ABC of Clinical Haematology* is to provide an overview of each disease area, with each chapter written by recognized experts in their respective areas. The structure of the book remains true to the original ABC ethos with succinct text and the liberal use of illustrations and photographic material. Key references providing more detailed information can be found at the end of each chapter to assist readers who may wish to obtain more detailed information about particular topics.

The topics covered are similar to previous editions but several chapters have been rewritten by new authors. These include myelodysplasia, leukaemias and transplantation, lymphomas, as well as bleeding disorders. Other chapters have been extensively overhauled and new co-authors included to ensure that the content is fresh and up to date. The book should be of value to a wide variety of readers including medical students, nurses, family doctors, and other health professionals involved in the care of patients with haematological disorders.

Of course, the quality of the content and the writing are key factors in the success of a book such as this and I am indebted to my haematology colleagues who have contributed high quality chapters to the book.

I would also like to thank Eleanor Lines and Vicki Donald for their help and patience during the preparation of the material.

There may be errors or omissions, and I would welcome any comments concerning the book. Readers may also have suggestions for the next edition. I would very much like to hear these and can be contacted at a.b.provan@qmul.ac.uk.

Drew Provan

CHAPTER 1

Iron Deficiency Anaemia

Drew Provan

OVERVIEW

- Iron deficiency is the commonest cause of anaemia worldwide
- Iron deficiency is usually easily diagnosed from the red cell indices
- A drop in haemoglobin is generally a late feature of iron deficiency
- The serum ferritin is a reliable means of confirming the diagnosis but may be falsely normal or even elevated as a reactive phenomenon as ferritin is an acute phase protein
- Iron deficiency is not a diagnosis in itself and in males and postmenopasual women blood loss from the gastrointestinal tract must be excluded
- Oral iron is preferred for iron replacement therapy, but occasionally parenteral iron is required

Box 1.1 Risk factors for development of iron deficiency

- **Age:** infants (especially if there is a history of prematurity); adolescents; postmenopausal women; elderly people
- **Sex:** increased risk in women
- **Reproduction:** menorrhagia
- **Renal:** haematuria (rarer cause)
- **Gastrointestinal tract:** appetite or weight changes; changes in bowel habit; bleeding from rectum/melaena; gastric or bowel surgery
- **Drug history:** especially aspirin and non-steroidal anti-inflammatories
- **Social history:** diet, especially vegetarians
- **Physiological:** pregnancy; infancy; adolescence; breastfeeding; age of weaning

Iron deficiency is the commonest cause of anaemia worldwide and is frequently seen in general practice. Iron deficiency anaemia is caused by defective synthesis of haemoglobin, resulting in red cells that are smaller than normal (microcytic) and contain reduced amounts of haemoglobin (hypochromic).

Iron metabolism

Iron has a pivotal role in many metabolic processes, and the average adult contains 3–5 g of iron, of which two-thirds is in the oxygen-carrying molecule haemoglobin.

A normal Western diet provides about 15 mg of iron daily, of which 5–10% is absorbed (~ 1 mg), principally in the duodenum and upper jejunum, where the acidic conditions help the absorption of iron in the ferrous form. Absorption is helped by the presence of other reducing substances, such as hydrochloric acid and ascorbic acid. The body has the capacity to increase its iron absorption in the face of increased demand, for example, in pregnancy, lactation, growth spurts and iron deficiency (Box 1.1).

Once absorbed from the bowel, iron is transported across the mucosal cell to the blood, where it is carried by the protein transferrin to developing red cells in the bone marrow. Iron stores comprise ferritin, a labile and readily accessible source of iron and haemosiderin, an insoluble form found predominantly in macrophages.

About 1 mg of iron a day is shed from the body in urine, faeces, sweat and cells shed from the skin and gastrointestinal tract. Menstrual losses of an additional 20 mg per month and the increased requirements of pregnancy (500–1000 mg) contribute to the higher incidence of iron deficiency in women of reproductive age (Table 1.1, Box 1.2).

Clinical features of iron deficiency

The symptoms accompanying iron deficiency depend on how rapidly the anaemia develops. In cases of chronic, slow blood loss, the body adapts to the increasing anaemia and patients can often tolerate extremely low concentrations of haemoglobin, for example, < 7.0 g/dL, with remarkably few symptoms. Most patients complain of increasing lethargy and dyspnoea. More unusual symptoms are headaches, tinnitus and taste disturbance.

Table 1.1 Daily dietary iron requirements

	Amount (mg)
Male	1
Adolescence	2–3
Female (reproductive age)	2–3
Pregnancy	3–4
Infancy	1
Maximum bioavailability from normal diet	~4

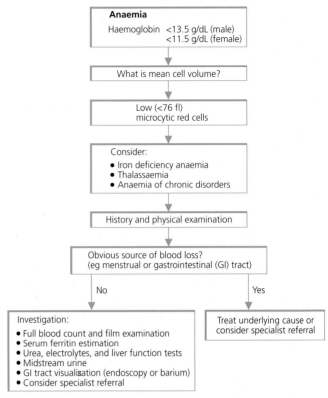

Figure 1.2 Diagnosis and investigation of iron deficiency anaemia.

On examination, several skin, nail and other epithelial changes may be seen in chronic iron deficiency. Atrophy of the skin occurs in about a third of patients and (rarely nowadays) nail changes such as koilonychia (spoon-shaped nails; Fig. 1.1) may result in brittle, flattened nails. Patients may also complain of angular stomatitis, in which painful cracks appear at the angle of the mouth, sometimes accompanied by glossitis. Although uncommon, oesophageal and pharyngeal webs can be a feature of iron deficiency anaemia (consider this in middle aged women presenting with dysphagia). These changes are believed to be due to a reduction in the iron-containing enzymes in the epithelium and gastrointestinal tract. Few of these epithelial changes are seen in modern practice, and they are of limited diagnostic value.

Tachycardia and cardiac failure may occur with severe anaemia irrespective of cause and, in such cases, prompt remedial action should be taken.

When iron deficiency is confirmed, a full clinical history, including leading questions on possible gastrointestinal blood loss or malabsorption (as in, for example, coeliac disease), should be obtained. Menstrual losses should be assessed and the importance of dietary factors and regular blood donation should not be overlooked (Fig. 1.2).

Diet alone is seldom the sole cause of iron deficiency anaemia in the UK except when it prevents an adequate response to a physiological challenge, as in pregnancy, for example.

Laboratory investigations

A full blood count and film should be assessed (Box 1.3). These will confirm the anaemia; recognizing the indices of iron deficiency is usually straightforward (reduced haemoglobin concentration, reduced mean cell volume, reduced mean cell haemoglobin, reduced mean cell haemoglobin concentration) (Table 1.2). Some modern analysers will determine the percentage of hypochromic red cells, which may be high before the anaemia develops (it is worth noting that a reduction in haemoglobin concentration is a late feature of iron deficiency). The blood film shows microcytic hypochromic red cells (Fig. 1.3). Hypochromic anaemia occurs in other disorders, such as anaemia of chronic disorders and sideroblastic anaemias,

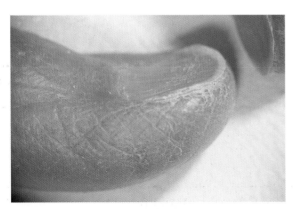

Figure 1.1 Nail changes in iron deficiency anaemia (koilonychia).

Box 1.3 **Investigations in iron deficiency anaemia**

- Full clinical history and physical examination
- Full blood count and blood film examination
- Haematinic assays (serum ferritin, vitamin B$_{12}$, folate)
- Note serum iron and TIBC now obsolete
- Percentage of hypochromic red cells and soluble transferrin receptor assay (if available)
- Urea and electrolytes, liver function tests
- Fibreoptic and/or barium studies of the gastrointestinal tract
- Pelvic ultrasound (female patients, if indicated)

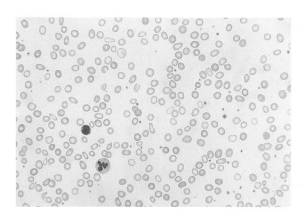

Figure 1.3 Blood film showing changes of iron deficiency anaemia.

and in globin synthesis disorders, such as thalassaemia (Table 1.3). To help to differentiate the type, further haematinic assays may be necessary. Historically, serum iron and total iron binding capacity (TIBC) were used in the diagnosis of iron deficiency anaemia, but because of the wide diurnal variation seen in iron levels and the lack of sensitivity, these assays are seldom used today. Difficulties in diagnosis arise when more than one type of anaemia is present, for example, iron deficiency and folate deficiency in malabsorption, in a population where thalassaemia is present, or in pregnancy, when the interpretation of red cell indices may be difficult.

Haematinic assays will demonstrate reduced serum ferritin concentration in straightforward iron deficiency. As an acute phase protein, however, the serum ferritin concentration may be normal or even raised in inflammatory or malignant disease.

A prime example of this is found in rheumatoid disease, in which active disease may result in a spuriously raised serum ferritin concentration masking an underlying iron deficiency caused by gastrointestinal bleeding after non-steroidal analgesic treatment. There may also be confusion in liver disease, as the liver contains stores of ferritin that are released after hepatocellular damage, leading to raised serum ferritin concentrations. In cases where ferritin estimation is likely to be misleading, the soluble transferrin receptor (sTfR) assay may aid the diagnosis.

Transferrin receptors are found on the surface of red cells in greater numbers in iron deficiency; a proportion of receptors is shed into the plasma and can be measured using commercial kits. Unlike serum ferritin, the level of sTfR does not rise in inflammatory disorders, and

Table 1.2 Diagnosis of iron deficiency anaemia

Reduced haemoglobin	Men <13.5 g/dl, women <11.5 g/dl
Reduced MCV	<76 fl (76–95 fl)
Reduced MCH	29.5 ± 2.5 pg (27.0–32.0 pg)
Reduced MCHC	32.5 ± 2.5 g/dl (32.0–36.0 g/dl)
Blood film	Microcytic hypochromic red cells with pencil cells and target cells
Reduced serum ferritin*	Men <10 μg/L, women (postmenopausal) <10 μg/L (premenopausal) <5 μg/L
Elevated % hypochromic red cells (>2%)	
Elevated soluble transferrin receptor level	

*Check with local laboratory for reference ranges. Note normal values in parentheses
MCH, mean corpuscular haemoglobin; MCHC, mean corpuscular haemoglobin concentration; MCV, mean corpuscular volume

Table 1.3 Characteristics of anaemia associated with other disorders

	Iron deficiency	Chronic disorders	Thalassaemia trait (α or β)	Sideroblastic anaemia
Degree of anaemia	Any	Seldom <9.0 g/dl	Mild	Any
MCV	↓	N or ↓	↓↓	N or ↓ or ↑
Serum ferritin	↓	N or ↑	N	↑
sTfR	↑	N	↑	N
Marrow iron	Absent	Present	Present	Present

MCV, mean corpuscular volume; N, normal; sTfR, soluble transferrin receptor assay hence can help to differentiate between anaemia due to inflammation and iron deficiency.

Diagnostic bone marrow sampling is seldom performed in simple iron deficiency, but, if the diagnosis is in doubt, a marrow aspirate may be carried out to demonstrate absent bone marrow stores.

When iron deficiency has been diagnosed, the underlying cause should be investigated and treated. Often the history will indicate the likely source of bleeding, for example, menstrual blood loss or gastrointestinal bleeding. If there is no obvious cause, further investigation generally depends on the age and sex of the patient. In male patients and postmenopausal women, possible gastrointestinal blood loss is investigated by visualization of the gastrointestinal tract (endoscopic or barium studies). Faecal occult blood tests are of no value in the investigation of iron deficiency.

Management

Effective management of iron deficiency relies on (i) the appropriate management of the underlying cause (for example, gastrointestinal or menstrual blood loss) and (ii) iron replacement therapy.

Oral iron replacement therapy, with gradual replenishment of iron stores and restoration of haemoglobin, is the preferred treatment. Oral ferrous salts are the treatment of choice (ferric salts are less well absorbed) and usually take the form of ferrous sulphate 200 mg three times daily (providing 65 mg × 3 = 195 mg elemental iron/day) (Fig. 1.4). Alternative preparations include ferrous gluconate and ferrous fumarate (Table 1.4). All three compounds, however, are associated with a high incidence of side effects, including nausea, constipation and diarrhoea. These side effects may be reduced by taking the tablets after meals, but even milder symptoms account for poor compliance with oral iron supplementation. It is worth noting that these lower gastrointestinal symptoms are not dose related. Modified release preparations have been developed to reduce side effects, but in practice prove expensive and often release the iron beyond the sites of optimal absorption.

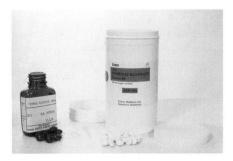

Figure 1.4 Oral iron replacement therapy.

Table 1.4 Elemental iron content of various oral iron preparations

Preparation	Amount (mg)	Ferrous iron (mg)
Ferrous fumarate	200	65
Ferrous gluconate	300	35
Ferrous sulphate	300	60

Effective iron replacement therapy should result in a rise in haemoglobin concentration of around 0.1 g/dL per day (about 2 g/dL every 3 weeks), but this varies from patient to patient. Once the haemoglobin concentration is within the normal range, iron replacement should continue for 3 months to replenish the iron stores.

Failure to respond to oral iron therapy

The main reason for failure to respond to oral iron therapy is poor compliance. However, if the losses (for example, bleeding) exceed the amount of iron absorbed daily, the haemoglobin concentration will not rise as expected; this will also be the case in combined deficiency states.

The presence of underlying inflammation or malignancy may also lead to a poor response to therapy. Occasionally, malabsorption of iron, such as that seen in coeliac disease, may lead to a failure to respond. Finally, an incorrect diagnosis of iron deficiency anaemia should be considered in patients who fail to respond adequately to iron replacement therapy.

Intravenous and intramuscular iron preparations

Parenteral iron may be used when the patient cannot tolerate oral supplements, for example, when patients have severe gastrointestinal side effects or if the losses exceed the daily amount that can be absorbed orally (Box 1.4). The rise in haemoglobin concentration is no faster with parenteral iron preparations than with oral iron therapy.

Intramuscular iron sorbitol (a complex of iron, sorbitol and citric acid) injection was used as a parenteral iron replacement for many years, but was discontinued in the UK in 2003. Generally, around 10–20 deep intramuscular injections were given over 2–3 weeks. However, side effects were common and included pain, skin staining at the site of injection and arthralgia. Newer intravenous iron preparations include iron hydroxide sucrose (Venofer®) and iron dextran (Cosmofer®, may also be given IM) for use in selected cases and under strict medical supervision, for example, on a haematology day unit (risk of anaphylaxis or other reactions).

Alternative treatments

Blood transfusion is not indicated unless the patient has decompensated due to a drop in haemoglobin concentration and needs a more rapid rise in haemoglobin, for example, in cases of worsening angina or severe coexisting pulmonary disease. In cases of iron deficiency with serious ongoing acute bleeding, blood transfusion may be required.

Prevention

When absorption from the diet is likely to be matched or exceeded by losses, extra sources of iron should be considered, for example,

> Box 1.4 **Intravenous iron preparations**
>
> - Intramuscular iron sorbitol no longer available (severe reactions)
> - Iron hydroxide sucrose and iron dextran are currently available in the UK
> - Useful in selected cases
> - Must be given under close medical supervision and where full resuscitation facilities are available
> - A test dose is recommended before administration of the full dose

prophylactic iron supplements in pregnancy or after gastrectomy, or encouragement of breastfeeding or use of formula milk during the first year of life (rather than cows' milk, which is a poor source of iron).

Further reading

Baer AN, Dessypris EN, Krantz SB. The pathogenesis of anemia in rheumatoid arthritis: a clinical and laboratory analysis. *Seminars in Arthritis and Rheumatism* 1990; **19**: 209–23.

Beguin Y. Soluble transferrin receptor for the evaluation of erythropoiesis and iron status. *Clinica Chimica Acta* 2003; **329**: 9–22.

Cook JD. Diagnosis and management of iron deficiencyanaemia. *Balliere's Best Practice and Research. Clinical Haematology* 2005; **18**: 319–32.

Cook JD, Skikne BS, Baynes RD. Iron deficiency: the global perspective. *Advances in Experimental Medicine and Biology* 1994; **356**: 219–28.

DeMaeyer E, Adiels-Tegman M. The prevalence of anaemia in the world. *World Health Statistics Quarterly* 1985; **38**: 302–16.

Demir A, Yarali N, Fisgin T *et al.* Serum transferrin receptor levels in beta-thalassemia trait. *Journal of Tropical Pediatrics* 2004; **50**: 369–71.

Ferguson BJ, Skikne BS, Simpson KM *et al.* Serum transferrin receptor distinguishes the anemia of chronic disease from iron deficiency anemia. *Journal of Laboratory and Clinical Medicine* 1992; **119**: 385–90.

Lozoff B, De Andraca I, Castillo M *et al.* Behavioral and developmental effects of preventing iron deficiency anemia in healthy full-term infants. *Pediatrics* 2003; **112**: 846–54.

McIntyre AS, Long RG. Prospective survey of investigations in outpatients referred with iron deficiency anaemia. *Gut* 1993; **34**: 1102–7.

Provan D. Mechanisms and management of iron deficiency anaemia. *British Journal of Haematology* 1999; **105**(Suppl 1): 19–26.

Punnonen K, Irjala K, Rajamaki A. Serum transferrin receptor and its ratio to serum ferritin in the diagnosis of iron deficiency. *Blood* 1997; **89**: 1052–7.

Rockey DC, Cello JP. Evaluation of the gastrointestinal tract in patients with iron deficiency anemia. *New England Journal of Medicine* 1993; **329**: 1691–5.

Windsor CW, Collis JL. Anaemia and hiatus hernia: experience in 450 patients. *Thorax* 1967; **22**(1): 73–8.

Acknowledgements

Drs AG Smith and A Amos provided the photographic material and the source of the detail in Table 1.4 is the *British National Formulary*, No 32(Sept), 1995.

CHAPTER 2

Macrocytic Anaemias

A Victor Hoffbrand, Drew Provan

OVERVIEW

- Macrocytic red cells (MCV greater than 95fl) may be associated with a megaloblastic or normoblastic bone marrow
- Deficiencies of either vitamin B_{12} or folate lead to defective DNA synthesis, megaloblastic changes in the bone marrow and many other cells
- The blood count indices and blood film features of B_{12} and folate deficiencies are identical and specific haematinic assays are required to differentiate between them
- Pernicious anaemia is the commonest cause of B_{12} deficiency in the UK
- Folate deficiency occurs in pregnancy, prematurity, chronic haemolysis and other high cell turnover states
- Vitamin B_{12} deficiency may lead to progressive neuropathy even in the absence of anaemia

---

Macrocytosis is a rise in the mean cell volume (MCV) of red cells above the normal range (in adults 80–95 fl). It is detected using a blood count, in which the MCV and other red cell indices are measured. The MCV is lower in children than in adults, with a normal mean of 70 fl at 1 year of age, rising by about 1 fl each year until it reaches the adult volume at puberty.

The causes of macrocytosis fall into two groups: (i) deficiency of vitamin B_{12} (cobalamin) or folate (or rarely abnormalities of their metabolism), in which the bone marrow is megaloblastic (Box 2.1) and (ii) other causes (Box 2.2), in which the bone marrow is usually normoblastic. In this chapter, the two groups are considered separately. The steps to diagnose the cause of macrocytosis and subsequently to manage it are then considered.

Megaloblastic bone marrow

Megaloblastic bone marrow is exemplified by developing red blood cells that are larger than normal, with nuclei that are more immature than the cytoplasm. The underlying mechanism is defective DNA synthesis.

Defects of vitamin B_{12} metabolism, for example, transcobalamin II deficiency, nitrous oxide anaesthesia, or of folate metabolism (such as methotrexate treatment), or rare inherited defects of DNA synthesis, may all cause megaloblastic anaemia.

Box 2.1 Causes of megaloblastic anaemia

Diet
- Vitamin B_{12} deficiency: vegan diet, poor quality diet
- Folate deficiency: poor quality diet, old age, poverty, synthetic diet without added folic acid, goats' milk

Malabsorption
- Gastric causes of vitamin B_{12} deficiency: pernicious anaemia, congenital intrinsic factor deficiency or abnormality, gastrectomy
- Intestinal causes of vitamin B_{12} deficiency: stagnant loop, congenital selective malabsorption, ileal resection, Crohn's disease
- Intestinal causes of folate deficiency: coeliac disease, tropical sprue, jejunal resection

Increased cell turnover
- Folate deficiency: pregnancy, prematurity, chronic haemolytic anaemia (such as sickle cell anaemia), extensive inflammatory and malignant diseases

Renal loss
- Folate deficiency: congestive cardiac failure, dialysis

Drugs
- Folate deficiency: anticonvulsants, sulphasalazine

Box 2.2 Other causes of macrocytosis*

- Alcohol
- Myelodysplasia
- Liver disease
- Cytotoxic drugs
- Hypothyroidism
- Paraproteinaemia (such as myeloma)
- Reticulocytosis
- Pregnancy
- Aplastic anaemia
- Neonatal period
- Red cell aplasia

*These are usually associated with a normoblastic marrow

Deficiency of vitamin B_{12} or folate

Vitamin B_{12} deficiency

The body's requirement for vitamin B_{12} is about 1 µg daily. This is

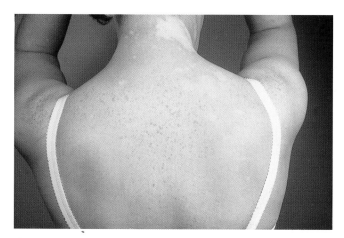

Figure 2.1 Patient with vitiligo on neck and back.

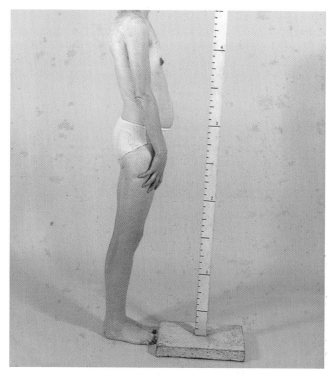

Figure 2.2 Patient with coeliac disease: underweight and low stature.

amply supplied by a normal Western diet (vitamin B$_{12}$ content 10–30 μg daily) but not by a strict vegan diet, which excludes all animal produce (including milk, eggs and cheese). Absorption of vitamin B$_{12}$ is through the ileum, facilitated by intrinsic factor, which is secreted by the parietal cells of the stomach. Absorption by this mechanism is limited to 2–3 μg daily.

In Britain, vitamin B$_{12}$ deficiency is usually due to pernicious anaemia, which now accounts for up to 80% of all cases of megaloblastic anaemia. The incidence of the disease is 1:10000 in northern Europe and the disease occurs in all races. The underlying mechanism is an autoimmune gastritis that results in achlorhydria and the absence of intrinsic factor. The incidence of pernicious anaemia peaks at 60 years of age; the condition has a female:male incidence of 1.6:1.0 and is more common in those with early greying of hair, blue eyes, blood group A and in those with a family history of pernicious anaemia or associated diseases, for example, vitiligo (Fig. 2.1), myxoedema, Hashimoto's disease, Addison's disease and hypoparathyroidism.

Other causes of vitamin B$_{12}$ deficiency are infrequent in the UK. A vegan lifestyle is an unusual cause of severe deficiency, as most vegetarians and vegans include some vitamin B$_{12}$ in their diet. Moreover, unlike in pernicious anaemia, the enterohepatic circulation for vitamin B$_{12}$ is intact in vegans, so vitamin B$_{12}$ stores are conserved. Gastric resection and intestinal causes of malabsorption of vitamin B$_{12}$, for example, ileal resection or the intestinal stagnant loop syndrome, are less common now that abdominal tuberculosis is infrequent and H2 antagonists have been introduced for treating peptic ulceration, thus reducing the need for gastrectomy.

Folate deficiency

The daily requirement for folate is 100–200 μg and a normal mixed diet contains about 200–300 μg. Natural folates are largely found in the polyglutamate form and these are absorbed through the upper small intestine after deconjugation and conversion to the monoglutamate 5-methyltetrahydrofolate.

Body stores are sufficient for only about 4 months. Folate deficiency may arise because of inadequate dietary intake, malabsorption (especially coeliac disease; Fig. 2.2), or excessive use caused by proliferating cells, which degrade folate. Deficiency in pregnancy may be due partly to inadequate diet, partly to transfer of folate to the fetus and partly to increased folate degradation.

Consequences of vitamin B$_{12}$ or folate deficiency
Megaloblastic anaemia

Clinical features include pallor and jaundice. The onset is gradual, and a severely anaemic patient may present with congestive heart failure or only when an infection supervenes. The blood film shows oval macrocytes and hypersegmented neutrophil nuclei (with six or more lobes) (Fig. 2.3). In severe cases, the white cell count and platelet count also fall (pancytopenia). The bone marrow shows characteristic megaloblastic erythroblasts and giant metamyelocytes (granulocyte precur-

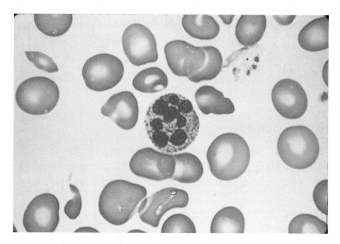

Figure 2.3 Blood film in vitamin B$_{12}$ deficiency showing macrocytic red cells and a hypersegmented neutrophil.

sors). Biochemically, there is an increase of unconjugated bilirubin and serum lactic dehydrogenase in the plasma, with, in severe cases, an absence of haptoglobins and presence of haemosiderin in the urine. These changes, including jaundice, are due to increased destruction of red cell precursors in the marrow (ineffective erythropoiesis).

Vitamin B$_{12}$ neuropathy

A minority of patients with vitamin B$_{12}$ deficiency develop a neuropathy due to symmetrical damage to the peripheral nerves and posterior and lateral columns of the spinal cord, the legs being more affected than the arms. Psychiatric abnormalities and visual disturbance may also occur. Men are more commonly affected than women. The neuropathy may occur in the absence of anaemia. Psychiatric changes and, at most, a mild peripheral neuropathy may be ascribed to folate deficiency.

Neural tube defects

Folic acid supplements in pregnancy have been shown to reduce the incidence of neural tube defects (spina bifida, encephalocoele and anencephaly) in the fetus, and may also reduce the incidence of cleft palate and harelip (Box 2.3). No clear relation exists between the incidence of these defects and any folate deficiency in the mother, although the lower the maternal red cell folate (and serum vitamin B$_{12}$) concentrations, even within the normal range, the more likely neural tube defects are to occur in the fetus. An underlying mechanism in a minority of cases is a genetic defect in folate metabolism, a mutation in the enzyme 5,10-methylene-tetrahydrofolate reductase. An autoantibody to folate receptors has been detected in pregnancy in some women who have babies with neural tube defects.

Gonadal dysfunction

Deficiency of either vitamin B$_{12}$ or folate may cause sterility, which is reversible with appropriate vitamin supplementation.

Epithelial cell changes

Glossitis may occur, and other epithelial surfaces may show cytological abnormalities (Fig. 2.4).

Box 2.3 Preventing folate deficiency in pregnancy

- As prophylaxis against folate deficiency in pregnancy, daily doses of folic acid 400 µg are usual
- Larger doses are not recommended as they could theoretically mask megaloblastic anaemia due to vitamin B$_{12}$ deficiency and thus allow B$_{12}$ neuropathy to develop
- As neural tube defects occur by the 28th day of pregnancy, it is advisable for a woman's daily folate intake to be increased by 400 µg/day at the time of conception
- The US Food and Drugs Administration announced in 1996 that specified grain products (including most enriched breads, flours, cornmeal, rice, noodles and macaroni) will be required to be fortified with folic acid to levels ranging from 0.43 mg to 1.5 mg per pound (453 g) of product. Fortification of flour with folic acid is currently under discussion in the UK
- For mothers who have already had an infant with a neural tube defect, larger doses of folic acid, for example, 5 mg daily, are recommended before and during subsequent pregnancy

---

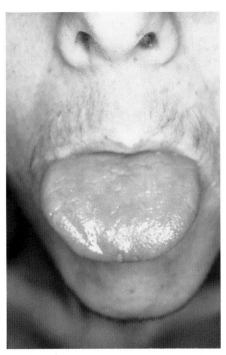

Figure 2.4 Glossitis due to vitamin B$_{12}$ deficiency.

Cardiovascular disease

Raised serum homocysteine concentrations have been associated with arterial obstruction (myocardial infarct, peripheral vascular disease or stroke) and venous thrombosis. Trials are under way to determine whether folic acid supplementation reduces the incidence of these vascular diseases.

Other causes of macrocytosis

The most common cause of macrocytosis in the UK is alcohol. Fairly small quantities of alcohol, for example, two gin and tonics or half a bottle of wine a day, especially in women, may cause a rise of MCV to >100 fl, typically without anaemia or any detectable change in liver function.

The mechanism for the rise in MCV is uncertain. In liver disease, the red cell volume may rise as a result of excessive lipid deposition on red cell membranes, and the rise is particularly pronounced in liver disease caused by alcohol. A modest rise in MCV is found in severe thyroid deficiency.

Physiological causes of macrocytosis are pregnancy and the neonatal period. In other causes of macrocytosis, other haematological abnormalities are usually present; in myelodysplasia (a frequent cause of macrocytosis in elderly people), there are usually quantitative or qualitative changes in the white cells and platelets in the blood. In aplastic anaemia, pancytopenia is present; pure red cell aplasia may also cause macrocytosis. Changes in plasma proteins, for example, presence of a paraprotein (as in myeloma), may cause a rise in MCV without macrocytes being present in the blood film. Drugs that affect DNA synthesis, for example, hydroxyurea and azathioprine, can cause macrocytosis with or without megaloblastic changes. Finally, a rare, benign familial type of macrocytosis has been described.

Diagnosis

Biochemical assays

The most widely used screening tests for the deficiencies are the serum vitamin B_{12} and folate assays (Box 2.4). A low serum concentration implies deficiency, but a subnormal serum concentration may occur in the absence of pronounced body deficiency, for example, in pregnancy (vitamin B_{12}) and with recent poor dietary intake (folate).

Red cell folate can also be used to screen for folate deficiency; a low concentration usually implies appreciable depletion of body folate, but the concentration also falls in severe vitamin B_{12} deficiency, and so it is more difficult to interpret the significance of a low red cell count than serum folate concentration in patients with megaloblastic anaemia. Moreover, if the patient has received a recent blood transfusion, the red cell folate concentration will partly reflect the folate concentration of the transfused red cells.

Specialist investigations

Assays of serum homocysteine (raised in vitamin B_{12} or folate deficiency) or methylmalonic acid (raised in vitamin B_{12} deficiency) are used in some specialized laboratories. Serum homocysteine levels are also raised in renal failure and with certain drugs, such as corticosteroids, and they increase with age and smoking.

Autoantibodies

For patients with vitamin B_{12} or folate deficiency, it is important to establish the underlying cause. In pernicious anaemia, intrinsic factor antibodies are present in plasma in 50% of patients and in parietal cell antibodies in 90%. Antiendomysial and antitransglutaminase antibodies are usually positive in coeliac disease.

Other investigations

A bone marrow examination is usually performed to confirm megaloblastic anaemia (Fig. 2.5). It is also required for the diagnosis of myelodysplasia (Fig. 2.6), aplastic anaemia, myeloma, or other marrow disorders associated with macrocytosis.

> Box 2.4 **Investigations that may be needed in patients with macrocytosis**
>
> - Serum vitamin B_{12} assay
> - Serum and red cell folate assays
> - Liver and thyroid function
> - Reticulocyte count
> - Serum protein electrophoresis
> - For vitamin B_{12} deficiency: serum parietal cell and intrinsic factor antibodies, radioactive vitamin B_{12} absorption with and without intrinsic factor (Schilling's test), possibly serum gastrin concentration
> - For folate deficiency: antiendomysial and antitransglutaminase antibodies
> - Consider bone marrow examination for megaloblastic changes suggestive of vitamin B_{12} or folate deficiency, or alternative diagnoses, for example, myelodysplasia, aplastic anaemia, myeloma
> - Endoscopy: gastric biopsy (vitamin B_{12} deficiency); duodenal biopsy (folate deficiency)

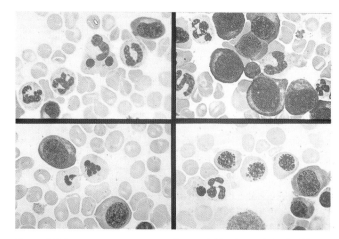

Figure 2.5 Bone marrow appearances in megaloblastic anaemia: developing red cells are larger than normal, with nuclei that are immature relative to their cytoplasm (nuclear : cytoplasmic asynchrony).

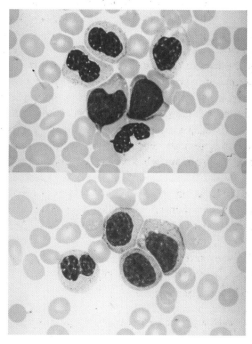

Figure 2.6 Bone marrow aspirate in myelodysplasia showing characteristic dysplastic neutrophils with bilobed nuclei. Reproduced with permission from *Clinical Haematology* (AV Hoffbrand, J Pettit), 3rd edn. St Louis: CV Mosby, 2000.

Radioactive vitamin B_{12} absorption studies, for example, Schilling's test, show impaired absorption of the vitamin in pernicious anaemia (Table 2.1); this can be corrected by giving intrinsic factor. In patients with an intestinal lesion, however, absorption of vitamin B_{12} cannot be corrected with intrinsic factor. Human intrinsic factor is no longer licensed for this test because of concern about transmission of prion disease.

Endoscopy should be performed to confirm atrophic gastritis and exclude gastric carcinoma or gastric polyps, which are 2–3 times more common in patients with pernicious anaemia than in age- and sex-matched controls.

Table 2.1 Results of absorption tests of radioactive vitamin B_{12}

	Dose of vitamin B_{12} given alone	Dose of vitamin B_{12} given with intrinsic factor[†]
Vegan	Normal	Normal
Pernicious anaemia or gastrectomy	Low	Normal
Ileal resection	Low	Low
Intestinal blind loop syndrome	Low*	Low*

*Corrected by antibiotics.
†Human intrinsic factor no longer licensed for this test because of concern about prion transmission

If folate deficiency is diagnosed, it is important to assess dietary folate intake and to exclude coeliac disease by tests for serum antiendomysial and antitransglutaminase antibodies, endoscopy and duodenal biopsy. The deficiency is common in patients with diseases of increased cell turnover who also have a poor diet.

Treatment

Vitamin B_{12} deficiency is treated initially by giving the patient six injections of hydroxocobalamin 1 mg at intervals of about 3–4 days, followed by four such injections a year for life. For patients undergoing total gastrectomy or ileal resection, it is sensible to start the maintenance injections from the time of operation. For vegans, less frequent injections, for example, 1–2 per year, may be sufficient, and the patient should be advised to eat foods to which vitamin B_{12} has been added, such as certain fortified breads or other foods.

Folate deficiency is treated with folic acid, usually 5 mg daily orally for 4 months, which is continued only if the underlying cause cannot be corrected. As prophylaxis against folate deficiency in patients with a severe haemolytic anaemia, such as sickle cell anaemia, 5 mg folic acid once weekly is probably sufficient. Vitamin B_{12} deficiency must be excluded in all patients starting folic acid treatment at these doses, as such treatment may correct the anaemia in vitamin B_{12} deficiency but allow neurological disease to develop.

Further reading

Carmel R. Current concepts in cobalamin deficiency. *Annual Reviews in Medicine* 2000; 51: 357–75.

Clarke R, Grimley Evans J, Schneede J *et al.* Vitamin B12 and folate deficiency in later life. *Age and Ageing* 2004; **33**: 34–41.

Hershko C, Hoffbrand AV, Keret D *et al.* Role of autoimmune gastritis, Helicobacter pylori and celiac disease in refractory or unexplained iron deficiency anemia. *Haematologica* 2005; **90**: 585–95.

Jacques PF, Selhub J, Bostom AG *et al.* The effect of folic acid fortification on plasma folate and total homocysteine concentrations. *New England Journal of Medicine* 1999; **340**: 1449–54.

Lindenbaum J, Allen RH. Clinical spectrum and diagnosis of folate deficiency. In: Bailey LB, ed. *Folate in Health and Disease.* Marcel Dekker, New York, 1995, 43–73.

Mills JL. Fortification of foods with folic acid—how much is enough? *New England Journal of Medicine* 2000; **342**(19): 1442–5.

Perry DJ. Hyperhomocysteinaemia. *Bailliere's Best Practice and Research. Clinical Haematology* 1999; **12**: 451–77.

Rothenberg SP, da Costa MP, Sequeira JM *et al.* Autoantibodies against folate receptors in women with a pregnancy complicated by a neural-tube defect. *New England Journal of Medicine* 2004; **350**: 134–42.

Solomon LR. Cobalamin-responsive disorders in the ambulatory care setting: unreliability of cobalamin, methylmalonic acid, and homocysteine testing. *Blood* 2005; **105**: 978–85.

Wickramasinghe SN. Megaloblastic anaemia. *Bailliere's Clinical Haematology* 1995; **8**: 441–703.

CHAPTER 3

The Hereditary Anaemias

David J Weatherall

OVERVIEW

- Sickle cell anaemia occurs commonly in individuals from African, Middle Eastern and Indian populations
- Neonatal screening of appropriate populations can result in a significant decrease in mortality from sickle cell disease in early life. The beta thalassaemias also occur at a very high frequency in many tropical populations but are now encountered in every country
- Carrier detection, counselling and prenatal diagnosis has reduced the number of births of children with beta thalassaemia in many countries
- Carefully monitored treatment of serious forms of beta thalassaemia with transfusion and adequate chelation have greatly improved the prognosis
- The severe forms of alpha thalassaemia are restricted to the Far East and certain Mediterranean populations
- The homozygous state for the severe forms of alpha thalassaemia results in stillbirth and a high frequency of obstetric complications

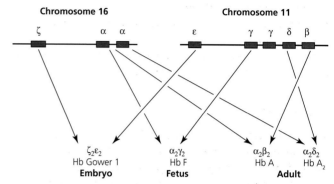

Figure 3.1 Simplified representation of the genetic control of human haemoglobin (Hb). Because α chains are shared by both fetal and adult Hb, mutations of the α globin genes affect Hb production in both fetal and adult life; diseases that are due to defective β globin production are only manifest after birth when Hb A replaces Hb F.

Box 3.1 **Sickling syndromes**

- Hb SS (sickle cell anaemia)
- Hb SC disease
- Hb S/β$^+$ thalassaemia
- Hb S/β$^°$ thalassaemia
- Hb SD disease

Hereditary anaemias include disorders of the structure or synthesis of haemoglobin (Hb), deficiencies of enzymes that provide the red cell with energy or protect it from chemical damage and abnormalities of the proteins of the red cell's membrane. Inherited diseases of haemoglobin (haemoglobinopathies) are by far the most important.

The structure of human Hb changes during development (Fig. 3.1). By the 12th week of gestation, embryonic haemoglobin is replaced by fetal haemoglobin (Hb F), which is slowly replaced after birth by the adult haemoglobins, Hb A and Hb A$_2$. Each type of haemoglobin consists of two different pairs of peptide chains; Hb A has the structure α$_2$β$_2$ (namely, two α chains plus two β chains), Hb A$_2$ has the structure α$_2$δ$_2$ and Hb F, α$_2$γ$_2$.

The haemoglobinopathies consist of structural haemoglobin variants (the most important of which are the sickling disorders) and thalassaemias (hereditary defects of the synthesis of either the α or β globin chains).

The sickling disorders

Classification and inheritance

The common sickling disorders consist of the homozygous state for the sickle cell gene, that is, sickle cell anaemia (Hb SS), and the compound heterozygous state for the sickle cell gene and for either Hb C (another β chain variant) or β thalassaemia (termed Hb SC disease or sickle cell β thalassaemia) (Box 3.1). The sickle cell mutation results in a single amino acid substitution in the β globin chain; heterozygotes have one normal (β^A) and one affected (β^S) β chain gene and produce about 60% Hb A and 40% Hb S; homozygotes produce mainly Hb S with small amounts of Hb F. Compound heterozygotes for Hb S and Hb C produce almost equal amounts of each variant, whereas those who inherit the sickle cell gene from one parent and β thalassaemia from the other make predominantly sickle haemoglobin (Fig. 3.2).

Pathophysiology

The amino acid substitution in the β globin chain causes red cell sickling during deoxygenation, leading to increased rigidity and aggregation in the microcirculation. These changes are reflected by a haemolytic anaemia and episodes of tissue infarction (Fig. 3.3).

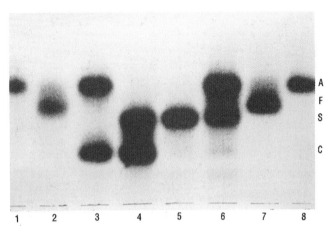

Figure 3.2 Haemoglobin electrophoresis showing (1) normal, (2) newborn, (3) Hb C trait (A-C), (4) Hb SC disease (SC), (5) sickle cell disease (SS), (6) sickle cell trait (A-S), (7) newborn, (8) normal.

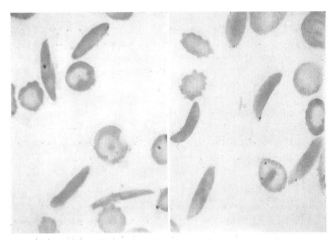

Figure 3.3 Peripheral blood film from patient with sickle cell anaemia showing sickled erythrocytes.

Box 3.2 **Sickle cell trait (Hb A and Hb S)**

- Less than half the Hb in each red cell is Hb S
- Occasional renal papillary necrosis
- Inability to concentrate the urine (older individuals)
- Red cells do not sickle unless oxygen saturation is <40% (rarely reached in venous blood)
- Painful crises and splenic infarction have been reported in severe hypoxia, such as in unpressurized aircraft, or under anaesthesia
- Sickling is more severe where Hb S is present with another β globin chain abnormality, such as Hb S and Hb C (Hb SC) or Hb S and Hb D (Hb SD)

Geographical distribution

The sickle cell gene is spread widely throughout Africa and in countries with African immigrant populations; some Mediterranean countries, the Middle East and parts of India. Screening should not be restricted to people of African origin.

Clinical features

Sickle cell carriers are not anaemic and have no clinical abnormalities (Box 3.2). Patients with sickle cell anaemia have a haemolytic anaemia, with a low haemoglobin concentration and a high reticulocyte count; the blood film shows polychromasia and sickled erythrocytes (Fig. 3.3, Box 3.3).

Patients adapt well to their anaemia and it is the vascular occlusive or sequestration episodes ('crises') that pose the main threat (Box 3.4). Crises take several forms. The commonest, called the painful crisis, is associated with widespread bone pain and is usually self-limiting. More serious and life-threatening crises include the sequestration of red cells into the lung or spleen, strokes, or red cell aplasia associated with parvovirus infections.

Diagnosis

Sickle cell anaemia should be suspected in any patient of an appro-

Box 3.3 **Sickle cell anaemia (homozygous Hb S)**

- Anaemia (Hb 6.0–10.0 g/dL): symptoms milder than expected as Hb S has reduced oxygen affinity (that is, gives up oxygen to tissues more easily)
- Sickled cells may be present in blood film: sickling occurs at oxygen tensions found in venous blood; cyclical sickling episodes
- Reticulocytes: raised to 10–20%
- Red cells contain ≥80% Hb S (rest is fetal Hb)
- Variable haemolysis
- Hand and foot syndrome (dactylitis)
- Intermittent episodes, or crises, characterized by bone pain, worsening anaemia, or pulmonary or neurological disease
- Chronic leg ulcers
- Gallstones

Box 3.4 **Complications of sickle cell disease**

- Hand and foot syndrome: seen in infancy; painful swelling of digits
- Painful crises: later in life; generalized bone pain; precipitated by cold, dehydration but often no cause found; self-limiting over a few days
- Aplastic crisis: marrow temporarily hypoplastic; may follow parvovirus infection; profound anaemia; reduced reticulocyte count
- Splenic sequestration crisis: common in infancy; progressive anaemia; enlargement of spleen
- Hepatic sequestration crisis: similar to splenic crisis but with sequestration of red cells in liver
- Lung or brain syndromes: sickling of red cells in pulmonary or cerebral circulation and endothelial damage to cerebral vessels in cerebral circulation
- Infections: particularly *Streptococcus pneumoniae* and *Haemophilus influenzae*
- Gallstones
- Progressive renal failure
- Chronic leg ulcers
- Recurrent priapism
- Aseptic necrosis of humoral/femoral head
- Chronic osteomyelitis: sometimes due to *Salmonella typhi*

priate racial group with a haemolytic anaemia. It can be confirmed by a sickle cell test, although this does not distinguish between heterozygotes and homozygotes. A definitive diagnosis requires haemoglobin electrophoresis and the demonstration of the sickle cell trait in both parents.

Prevention and treatment

Pregnant women in at-risk racial groups should be screened in early pregnancy and, if the woman and her partner are carriers, should be offered either prenatal or neonatal diagnosis. As soon as the diagnosis is established, babies should receive penicillin daily and be immunized against *Streptococcus pneumoniae*, *Haemophilus influenzae* type b and *Neisseria meningitidis*. Parents should be warned to seek medical advice on any suspicion of infection. Painful crises should be managed with adequate analgesics, hydration and oxygen. The patient should be observed carefully for a source of infection and a drop in haemoglobin concentration. Pulmonary sequestration crises require urgent exchange transfusion together with oxygen therapy. Strokes should be treated with an exchange transfusion; there is now good evidence that they can be prevented by regular surveillance of cerebral blood flow by Doppler examination and prophylactic transfusion. There is also good evidence that the frequency of painful crises can be reduced by maintaining patients on hydroxyurea, although, because of the uncertainty about the long-term effects of this form of therapy, it should be restricted to adults or, if it is used in children, should be used only for a short period. Aplastic crises require urgent blood transfusion. Splenic sequestration crises require transfusion and, because they may recur, splenectomy is advised (Box 3.5).

Sickling variants

Hb SC disease is characterized by a mild anaemia and fewer crises. Important microvascular complications, however, include retinal damage and blindness, aseptic necrosis of the femoral heads and recurrent haematuria. The disease is occasionally complicated by pulmonary embolic disease, particularly during and after pregnancy; these episodes should be treated by immediate exchange transfusion. Patients with Hb SC should have annual ophthalmological surveillance; the retinal vessel proliferation can be controlled with

Box 3.5 **Treatment of major complications of sickle cell disease**

- Hand and foot syndrome: hydration; paracetamol
- Painful crises: hydration; analgesia (including graded intravenous analgesics); oxygen (check arterial blood gases); blood cultures; antibiotics
- Pulmonary infiltrates: especially with deterioration in arterial gases, falling platelet count and/or haemoglobin concentration suggesting lung syndrome requires urgent exchange blood transfusion to reduce Hb S level together with oxygenation
- Splenic sequestration crisis: transfusion; splenectomy to prevent recurrence
- Neurological symptoms: immediate exchange transfusion followed by long-term transfusion
- Prevention of crises: ongoing trials of cytotoxic agent hydroxyurea show that it raises Hb F level and ameliorates frequency and severity of crises; long-term effects unknown

laser treatment. The management of the symptomatic forms of sickle cell β thalassaemia is similar to that of sickle cell anaemia.

The thalassaemias

Classification

The thalassaemias are classified as α or β thalassaemias, depending on which pair of globin chains is synthesized inefficiently. Rarer forms affect both β and δ chain production: δβ thalassaemias.

Distribution

The disease is broadly distributed throughout parts of Africa, the Mediterranean region, the Middle East, the Indian subcontinent and South East Asia, and it occurs sporadically in all racial groups (Fig. 3.4). Like sickle cell anaemia, it is thought to be common because the mutation protects carriers against malaria.

Inheritance

The β thalassaemias result from over 150 different mutations of the β globin genes, which reduce the output of β globin chains, either

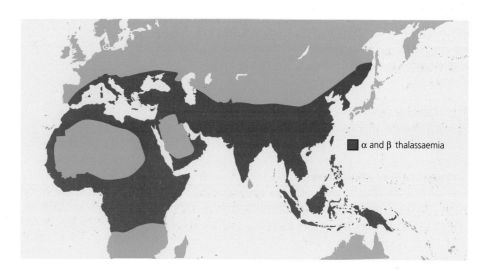

Figure 3.4 Distribution of the thalassaemias (red area).

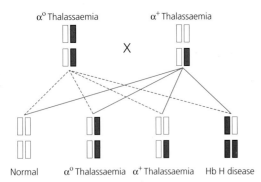

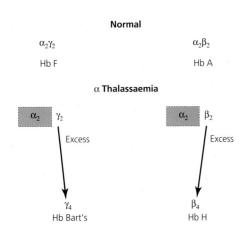

Figure 3.5 Inheritance of Hb disease (open boxes represent normal α globin genes and red boxes deleted α globin genes).

Normal

$\alpha_2\gamma_2$ $\alpha_2\beta_2$

Hb F   Hb A

α Thalassaemia

α_2 γ_2 α_2 β_2

Excess   Excess

γ_4 β_4

Hb Bart's   Hb H

High oxygen affinity, anoxia unstable, haemolysis

Figure 3.6 Pathophysiology of α thalassaemia.

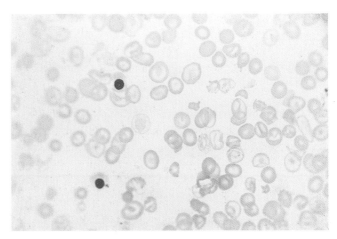

Figure 3.7 Peripheral blood film in homozygous β thalassaemia showing pronounced hypochromia and anisocytosis with nucleated red blood cells.

Box 3.6 β **Thalassaemia trait (heterozygous carrier)**

- Mild hypochromic microcytic anaemia
- Haemoglobin 9.0–11.0 g/dL
- Mean cell volume 5.0–7.0 g/dL
- Mean corpuscular haemoglobin 20–22 pg
- No clinical features, patients asymptomatic
- Occasional symptomatic anaemia in pregnancy
- Often diagnosed on routine blood count
- Raised Hb A_2 level

Box 3.7 β **Thalassaemia major (homozygous β thalassaemia)**

- Severe anaemia
- Blood film
  - Pronounced variation in red cell size and shape
  - Pale (hypochromic) red cells
  - Target cells
  - Basophilic stippling
  - Nucleated red cells
  - Moderately raised reticulocyte count
- Infants are well at birth but develop anaemia in first few months of life when switch occurs from γ to β globin chains
- Progressive splenomegaly; iron loading; susceptibility to infection

---

completely (β° thalassaemia) or partially (β⁺ thalassaemia). They are inherited in the same way as sickle cell anaemia; carrier parents have a one in four chance of having a homozygous child. The genetics of the α thalassaemias is more complicated because normal people have two α globin genes on each of their chromosomes 16. If both are lost (α° thalassaemia) no α globin chains are made, whereas if only one of the pair is lost (α⁺ thalassaemia) the output of α globin chains is reduced (Fig. 3.5). Impaired α globin production leads to excess γ or β chains that form unstable and physiologically useless tetramers: γ_4 (Hb Bart's) and β_4 (Hb H) (Fig. 3.6). The homozygous state for α° thalassaemia results in the Hb Bart's hydrops syndrome, whereas the inheritance of α° and α⁺ thalassaemia produces Hb H disease.

The β thalassaemias

Heterozygotes for β thalassaemia are asymptomatic, have hypochromic microcytic red cells with a low mean cell haemoglobin and mean cell volume (Fig. 3.7), and have a mean Hb A_2 level of about twice that of normal (Box 3.6). Homozygotes, or those who have inherited a different β thalassaemia gene from both parents, usually develop severe anaemia in the first year of life (Box 3.7). This results from a deficiency of β globin chains; excess α chains precipitate in the red cell precursors leading to their damage, either in the bone marrow or

the peripheral blood. Hypertrophy of the ineffective bone marrow leads to skeletal changes, and there is variable hepatosplenomegaly. The Hb F level is always raised. If these children are transfused, the marrow is 'switched off', and growth and development may be normal. However, they accumulate iron and may die later from damage to the myocardium, pancreas, or liver (Fig. 3.8). They are also prone to infection and folic acid deficiency.

Milder forms of β thalassaemia (thalassaemia intermedia), although not transfusion dependent, are often associated with similar bone changes, anaemia, leg ulcers and delayed development. The most important form of β thalassaemia intermedia is Hb E β thalassaemia, which results from the inheritance of Hb E and a β thalassaemia

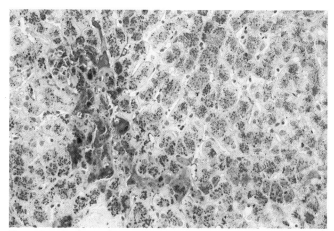

Figure 3.8 Liver biopsy from patient with β thalassaemia showing pronounced iron accumulation.

gene. This condition is the commonest form of severe thalassaemia in many parts of Asia and is associated with a remarkably diverse clinical course; some patients are transfusion dependent while others may remain asymptomatic.

The α thalassaemias

The Hb Bart's hydrops fetalis syndrome is characterized by the stillbirth of a severely oedematous (hydropic) fetus in the second half of pregnancy. Hb H disease is associated with a moderately severe haemolytic anaemia. The carrier states for $α^o$ thalassaemi a and the homozygous state for $α^+$ thalassaemia result in a mild hypochromic anaemia with normal Hb A_2 levels (Box 3.8). They can only be distinguished with certainty by DNA analysis in a specialized laboratory. In addition to the distribution mentioned above, α thalassaemia is also seen in European populations in association with mental retardation; the molecular pathology is quite different to the common inherited forms of the condition. There are two major forms of α thalassaemia associated with mental retardation (ATR); one is encoded on chromosome 16 (ATR-16) and the other on the X chromosome (ATR-X). ATR-16 is usually associated with mild mental retardation and is due to loss of the β globin genes together with other genetic material from the end of the short arm of chromosome 16. ATR-X is associated with more severe mental retardation and a variety of skeletal deformities, and is encoded by a gene on the X chromosome, which is expressed widely in different tissues during different stages of development. These conditions should be suspected in any infant or child with retarded development who has the haematological picture of a mild α thalassaemia trait.

Prevention and treatment

As β thalassaemia is easily identified in heterozygotes, pregnant women of appropriate racial groups should be screened; if a woman is found to be a carrier, her partner should be tested and the couple counselled. Prenatal diagnosis by chorionic villus sampling can be carried out between the ninth and 13th weeks of pregnancy (Box 3.9).

Babies with β thalassaemia major should be observed very carefully regarding growth, activity and steady-state haemoglobin level.

Box 3.8 **The α thalassaemias**

$-α/αα$ 1α gene deleted
- Asymptomatic
- Minority show reduced mean cell volume (MCV) and mean corpuscular haemoglobin (MCH)

$-α/-α$ or $αα/--$ 2α genes deleted
- Haemoglobin is normal or slightly reduced
- Reduced MCV and MCH
- No symptoms

$--/-α$ 3α genes deleted, Hb H disease
- Chronic haemolytic anaemia
- Reduced α chain production with formation of $β_4$ tetramers ($β_4$ is termed Hb H)
- Hb H is unstable and precipitates in older red cells
- Haemoglobin is 7.0–11.0g/dL, although may be lower
- Reduced MCV and MCH
- Clinical features: jaundice, hepatosplenomegaly, leg ulcers, gallstones, folate deficiency

$--/--$ 4α genes deleted, Hb Bart's hydrops
- No α chains produced
- Mainly γ, forms tetramers ($γ_4$ = Hb Bart's)
- Intrauterine death or stillborn at 25–40weeks or dies soon after birth

$αα/αα$ represents 2α globin genes inherited from each parent. Changes due to α thalassaemia are present from birth, unlike in β thalassaemia

---

Box 3.9 **Women with thalassaemia**

- Women with the haematological features of thalassaemia trait with normal Hb A_2 levels should be referred to a centre able to identify the different forms of α thalassaemia
- Those with $α^o$ thalassaemia trait, if their partners are similarly affected, should be referred for prenatal diagnosis
- This is because the haemoglobin Bart's hydrops syndrome is associated with an increased risk of toxaemia of pregnancy and postpartum bleeding due to a hypertrophied placenta

---

When it is certain that they require regular transfusion, they should be given washed red cell transfusions at monthly intervals; it is vital that the blood is screened for human immunodeficiency virus/acquired immunodeficiency syndrome, hepatitis B and C viruses and, in some countries, malaria.

To prevent iron overload, overnight infusions of desferrioxamine together with vitamin C should be started, and the patient's serum ferritin, or better, hepatic iron concentrations, should be monitored; complications of desferrioxamine include infections with *Yersinia* spp., retinal and acoustic nerve damage and reduction in growth associated with calcification of the vertebral discs.

The place of the oral chelating agent deferiprone is still under evaluation. Although it appears not to maintain iron balance in up to 50% of patients, and it causes neutropenia and variably severe arthritis, recent work suggests that it may be more effective in removing iron from the heart than desferrioxamine; this observation requires confirmation in prospective studies. Another recently developed oral chelating agent, Exjade ® (ICL670), is still under investigation; preliminary studies suggest that it may have comparable activity to desferrioxamine in maintaining iron balance and that it is relatively non-toxic, although further studies are required to confirm that it does not have a deleterious effect on renal function. Bone marrow transplantation, if appropriate HLA-DR-matched siblings are available, may carry a good prognosis if carried out early in life. Treatment with agents designed to raise the production of Hb F is still at the experimental stage.

In β thalassaemia and Hb H disease, progressive splenomegaly or increasing blood requirements, or both, indicate that splenectomy may be beneficial. Patients who undergo splenectomy should be vaccinated against *S. pneumoniae*, *H. influenzae* and *N. meningitidis* preoperatively, and should receive a maintenance dose of oral penicillin indefinitely.

Red cell enzyme defects

Red cells have two main metabolic pathways, one burning glucose anaerobically to produce energy, the other generating reduced glutathione to protect against injurious oxidants. Many inherited enzyme defects have been described. Some of those of the energy pathway, for example, pyruvate kinase deficiency, cause haemolytic anaemia; any child with this type of anaemia from birth should be referred to a centre capable of analysing the major red cell enzymes.

Glucose-6-phosphate dehydrogenase deficiency (G6PD) involves the protective pathway. It affects millions of people worldwide, mainly the same racial groups as are affected by the thalassaemias. G6PD deficiency is sex linked and affects predominantly males (Box 3.10). It causes neonatal jaundice, sensitivity to broad (fava) beans and haemolytic responses to oxidant drugs.

Red cell membrane defects

The red cell membrane is a complex sandwich of proteins that are required to maintain the integrity of the cell. There are many inherited defects of the membrane proteins, some of which cause haemolytic anaemia. Hereditary spherocytosis is due to a structural change that makes the cells more leaky. It is particularly important to identify this disease because it can be 'cured' by splenectomy. There are many rare inherited varieties of elliptical or oval red cells, some associated

---

Box 3.10 Drugs causing haemolysis in patients with G6PD deficiency

Antimalarials
- Primiquine
- Pamaquine

Analgesics*
- Phenacetin
- Acetyl salicylic acid

Others
- Sulphonamides
- Nalidixic acid
- Dapsone

*Probably only at high doses

---

with chronic haemolysis and response to splenectomy. A child with chronic haemolytic anaemia with abnormally shaped red cells should always be referred for expert advice.

Other hereditary anaemias

Other anaemias with an important inherited component include Fanconi's anaemia (hypoplastic anaemia with skeletal deformities), Blackfan–Diamond anaemia (red cell aplasia) and several forms of congenital dyserythropoietic anaemia.

Further reading

Gordon-Smith EC. Disorders of red cell metabolism. In: Hoffbrand AV, Catovsky D & Tuddenham EGD, eds. *Postgraduate Haematology*, 5th edn, Blackwell Publishing, Oxford, 2005, 133–150.

Lal A, Vichinsky EP. Sickle cell disease. In: Hoffbrand AV, Catovsky D & Tuddenham EGD, eds. *Postgraduate Haematology*, 5th edn. Blackwell Publishing, Oxford, 2005, 104–118.

Steinberg MH, Forget BG, Higgs DR, Nagel RL. *Disorders of Haemoglobin*. Cambridge University Press, Cambridge, 2001.

Weatherall DJ. The thalassemias. In: Stamatayonnopoulos G, Perlmutter RM, Marjerus PW *et al.*, eds. *Molecular Basis of Blood Diseases*, 3rd edn. WB Saunders, Philadelphia, 2001, 186–226.

Weatherall DJ. Haemoglobin and the inherited disorders of globin synthesis. In: Hoffbrand AV, Catovsky D & Tuddenham EGD, eds. *Postgraduate Haematology*, 5th edn. Blackwell Publishing, Oxford, 2005, 85–103.

Weatherall DJ, Clegg JB. *The Thalassemia Syndromes*, 4th edn. Blackwell Publishing, Oxford, 2001.

CHAPTER 4

Polycythaemia, Essential Thrombocythaemia and Myelofibrosis

George S Vassiliou, Anthony R Green

OVERVIEW

- The myeloproliferative disorders (MPDs) comprise polycythaemia vera (PV), essential thombocythaemia (ET) and idiopathic myelofibrosis (IMF)
- They are closely related clonal blood disorders of haemopoietic stem cells
- Appropriately treated PV and ET are compatible with long-term survival, whereas life expectancy is significantly reduced in IMF
- Arterial and venous thromboses are the commonest causes of morbidity and mortality in MPDs
- A recently identified activating mutation in the tyrosine kinase JAK2 (JAK2 V617F) is believed to underlie the pathogenesis of the majority of cases of MPD
- The mainstay of treatment in PV is venesection to maintain the haematocrit below 0.45
- Thrombocytosis in high risk patients with ET or PV should be treated with cytoreductive drugs such as hydroxyurea
- MPDs have an inherent risk of progression to acute leukaemia, highest in IMF

Polycythaemia vera (PV), essential thrombocythaemia (ET) and idiopathic myelofibrosis (IMF), known collectively as the classic myeloproliferative disorders (MPDs), are clonal disorders originating from a neoplastic haemopoietic stem cell. They are most common in middle or older age, and share several features, including a potential to transform into acute leukaemia and into each other. Treatment of PV and ET can greatly influence prognosis, hence the importance of differentiating them from other conditions associated with polycythaemia or a raised platelet count (thrombocytosis), the prognosis and treatment of which are different. Myelofibrosis may arise *de novo* (IMF) or result from progression of PV or ET.

Recently, acquired activating mutations in the gene for the tyrosine kinase JAK2, leading to a valine to phenylalanine substitution at amino acid 617 (V617F), were identified in nearly all cases of PV and approximately half the cases of ET and IMF (Fig. 4.1). The abnormally active mutant JAK2 is thought to amplify signalling downstream of cytokine receptors and thus to have a central role in the pathogenesis of MPDs.

Polycythaemia

An elevation in packed cell volume (PCV) defines polycythaemia (Fig. 4.2). A raised PCV (> 0.51 in men, > 0.48 in women) needs to be confirmed on a specimen taken without prolonged venous stasis (tourniquet), and patients with a persistently raised PCV may

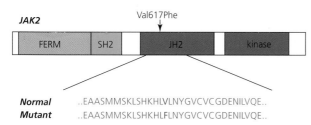

Figure 4.1 Diagrammatic representation of the JAK2 tyrosine kinase. The domain structure of the protein is outlined. The V617F (Val617Phe) substitution found in the majority of MPDs (arrow) disrupts the inhibitory pseudokinase domain (JH2) and leads to constitutive activation of the kinase.

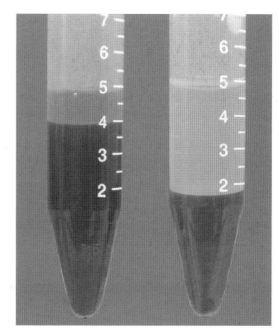

Figure 4.2 Raised pack cell volume (PCV) in a patient with polycythaemia vera (left) compared to a blood sample from a person with a normal PCV (right).

have to be investigated to exclude or confirm a diagnosis of PV (Fig. 4.1).

Estimation of total red cell mass or volume has been a key investigation in determining the cause of a raised PCV. Red cell mass is best expressed as the percentage difference between the measured value and that predicted for the patient's height and weight (derived from published tables). Red cell mass measurements >25% above the predicted value constitute true polycythaemia, which can be subclassified into aetiological categories (Box 4.1). When the PCV is raised but the red cell mass is not, the condition is known as apparent polycythaemia, and is secondary to a reduction in plasma volume. The role of red cell mass estimation is changing with the advent of molecular testing for JAK2 mutations.

Polycythaemia vera

Presentation can be incidental but is classically associated with a history of occlusive vascular lesions (stroke, transient ischaemic attack, ischaemic digits, venous thrombosis), headache, mental clouding, facial redness, itching, abnormal bleeding or gout.

Investigations

A raised white cell count ($> 10 \times 10^9$/L neutrophils) or a raised platelet count (>400×10^9/L) suggest primary polycythaemia, especially if both are raised in the absence of an obvious cause, such as infection or carcinoma. Serum ferritin concentration should be determined as iron deficiency may mask a raised PCV, resulting in a missed diagnosis of PV. If the spleen is not palpable, splenic size should be determined by ultrasonography.

Red cell mass should be measured to confirm true polycythaemia, unless a very high PCV (>0.60 in men or >0.56 in women) is present, as this invariably predicts a raised value (Box 4.2). Second-

ary polycythaemia should be excluded by confirming the absence of hypoxia and of a high serum erythropoietin concentration. Bone marrow cytogenetic analysis should be performed to identify acquired chromosomal abnormalities (Fig. 4.3). In addition, erythroid colony growth from blood in the absence of added erythropoietin culture from peripheral blood would support the diagnosis. However, this is a specialist test and not widely available. Finally, molecular testing for the JAK2 V617F mutation has rapidly become a key investigation, as it is present in most cases of PV. A proposed set of diagnostic criteria based on these investigations is outlined in Box 4.3. As the JAK2 mutation is present in the vast majority of cases, the diagnosis of PV is usually made on the basis of diagnostic criteria A1 + A2 + A4 (Box 4.3).

Treatment

Repeated venesection to maintain the PCV at < 0.45 has been shown to reduce the risk of thrombotic episodes in PV, as has the administration of low-dose aspirin (Box 4.4). Venesection has to be frequent at first, but is eventually needed only every 6–10 weeks in most patients. If thrombocytosis is present, concurrent therapy to maintain the platelet count to $< 400 \times 10^9$/L is necessary. Hydroxyurea (0.5–

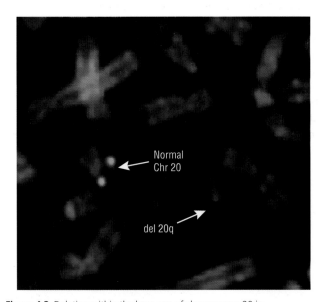

Figure 4.3 Deletion within the long arm of chromosome 20 in polycythaemia vera demonstrated by fluorescence *in situ* hybridization. ■, Probe for centromere of chromosome 20; ■, probe for part of long arm of chromosome 20.

1.5 g daily) is recommended for this purpose and is not thought to have a pronounced leukaemogenic potential. Some physicians use interferon-α in preference to hydroxyurea in younger patients, as this drug is theoretically even less likely to carry a leukaemogenic risk. Anagrelide can specifically reduce the platelet count but should be used with caution (see under Essential thrombocythaemia). Treatment with radioactive phosphorus (^{32}P) has been superseded because of the additional risk of inducing malignancies, including acute leukaemia, in later life, although oral busulfan may be a convenient drug in elderly patients.

Prognosis

Adequately treated patients with PV have a long median survival (> 10 years) but there is also a 20% incidence of transformation to myelofibrosis and 5% to acute leukaemia. The incidence of leukaemia is further increased in those who have transformed to myelofibrosis and in those treated with ^{32}P radiotherapy or multiple cytotoxic agents.

Secondary polycythaemia

Many causes of secondary polycythaemia have been identified, the commonest being chronic hypoxaemia and renal diseases, the kidneys being the site of erythropoietin production (Box 4.1). In recent years, the misuse of drugs such as erythropoietin and anabolic steroids has become a factor that also needs to be considered. Investigations aim to determine the underlying disorder to which the polycythaemia is secondary.

Treatment

Treatment is aimed at removing the underlying cause when practicable. In most cases of secondary polycythaemia, the risk of vascular occlusion is much less pronounced than in PV, and venesection is usually undertaken only in patients with a very high PCV. At this level, the harmful effects of increased viscosity outweigh the oxygen-carrying benefits of polycythaemia, and reduction to a PCV of 0.50–0.52 may result in an improved cardiopulmonary function. In practice, the symptoms experienced by individual patients often dictate the target PCV. In polycythaemia associated with renal lesions or other tumours, the PCV should generally be reduced to < 0.45.

Apparent polycythaemia

In apparent or relative polycythaemia, red cell mass is not increased and the raised PCV is secondary to a decrease in plasma volume. An association exists with smoking, alcohol excess, obesity, diuretics and hypertension.

Treatment

The need for treatment is uncertain. Lowering the PCV by venesection is undertaken only in patients who have a significantly increased risk of vascular complications for other reasons. On follow-up, up to one-third of patients spontaneously revert to a normal PCV.

Thrombocytosis

A raised platelet count (thrombocytosis) most commonly represents a reactive response to one or more of a diverse group of stimuli such as iron deficiency, inflammation or infection. Additionally, thrombocytosis can be due to one of several clonal blood disorders (Box 4.5).

Essential thrombocythaemia

A persisting platelet count > 600×10^9/L is the central diagnostic feature, but other reactive and clonal causes of a raised platelet count need to be excluded before a diagnosis of ET can be made. The diagnosis should not be missed, however, as, unlike reactive thrombocytosis, where the risk is small, ET carries a high risk of occlusive vascular events.

Laboratory investigations

The JAK2 V617F mutation is found in about half of cases with this disorder. In such cases, if PV and IMF can be ruled out, a diagnosis of ET can confidently be made. In the absence of JAK2 V617F, investigations will aim to exclude other causes of a raised platelet count. Apart from a full blood count and blood film, these investigations should include the erythrocyte sedimentation rate, serum C reac-

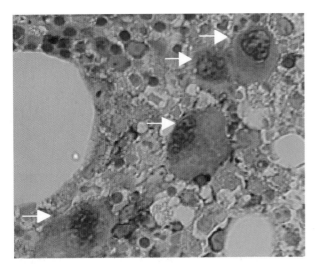

Figure 4.4 Bone marrow trephine biopsy from a patient with essential thrombocythaemia showing clustering of megakaryocytes (arrows).

tive protein, serum ferritin and bone marrow aspirate, trephine and cytogenetic analysis (Fig. 4.4). Trephine histology can often reveal features such as clusters of large megakaryocytes that are suggestive of ET, and although cytogenetics are generally normal in ET, certain abnormalities may favour a diagnosis of myelodysplasia or help to exclude a diagnosis of chronic myeloid leukaemia.

Presentation and prognosis

Between 30% and 50% of patients with ET have microvascular occlusive events, such as burning pain in the extremities (erythromelalgia) or digital ischaemia (Fig. 4.5), major vascular occlusive events, or haemorrhage at presentation. These are most pronounced in the elderly, in whom the risk of stroke, myocardial infarction or other vascular occlusion is high if left untreated. Patients with pre-existing vascular disease will also be at higher risk of such complications. The risk in young patients is lower, although major life-threaten-

ing events can still occur. In a minority of patients, transformation to myelofibrosis or acute leukaemia can occur, usually after many years.

Treatment and survival

All patients should receive daily low-dose aspirin, unless contraindicated because of allergy, bleeding or peptic ulceration. This reduces the risk of vascular occlusion but may increase the risk of haemorrhage, particularly at very high platelet counts.

Reduction of the platelet count with cytoreductive agents (daily hydroxyurea, or intermittent low-dose busulfan in elderly people) reduces the incidence of vascular complications and appreciably improves survival in older patients (from a median of about 3 years in untreated patients to 10 years or more in treated patients). Anagrelide is a platelet-specific agent, but as it appears to be less effective in reducing venous thromboses and to marginally increase the risk of transformation to myelofibrosis, it should be used as a second line agent. Interferon-α has also been used and is particularly useful in pregnancy.

Idiopathic myelofibrosis

The main features are bone marrow fibrosis, extramedullary haemopoiesis (production of blood cells in organs other than the bone marrow), splenomegaly and a leucoerythroblastic blood picture (immature red and white cells in the blood) (Fig. 4.6). Good evidence exists that the fibroblast proliferation is secondary and not part of the clonal process. In some patients, the fibrosis is accompanied by new bone formation (osteomyelosclerosis). IMF needs to be distinguished from causes of secondary myelofibrosis (see below).

Presentation

IMF can have a long pre-clinical period and, in some cases, patients may have had undiagnosed PV or ET. Although the diagnosis may be made in asymptomatic patients, the absence of a palpable spleen at presentation is rare. Usual presenting features are abdominal full-

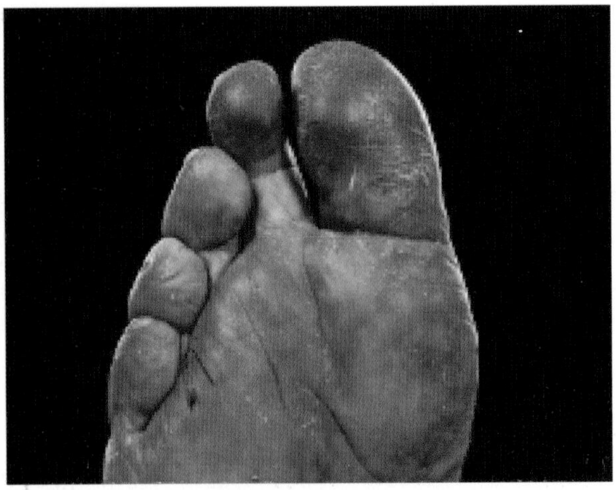

Figure 4.5 Toe ischaemia in a patient with essential thrombocythaemia.

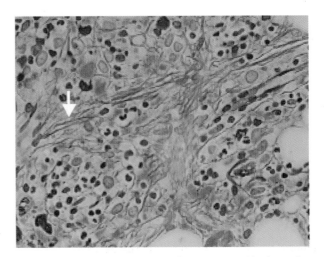

Figure 4.6 Bone marrow trephine biopsy from a patient with advanced idiopathic myelofibrosis. Note the marked linear reticulin staining (arrow).

ness or discomfort (splenomegaly), anaemia, fatigue and a bleeding diathesis. Fevers, night sweats and weight loss (hypermetabolic state) may be present and are associated with more advanced disease.

Laboratory investigations

Significant bone marrow fibrosis is the *sine qua non* of IMF. A leucoerythroblastic blood picture is characteristic but not diagnostic of IMF as it can occur in cases of marrow infiltration (e.g. by malignancy, amyloidosis, tuberculosis, osteopetrosis), severe sepsis, severe haemolysis and other circumstances (Box 4.6). The blood count in IMF is variable. In the initial 'proliferative phase', red cell production may be normal or even increased, and about half of presenting patients may have a raised white cell or platelet count (absence of the Philadelphia chromosome will distinguish from chronic myeloid leukaemia) (Fig. 4.7). However, as the bone marrow becomes more fibrotic, the more familiar 'cytopenic phase' supervenes. The JAK2 V617F mutation is found in about half of cases of IMF and can help to confirm the diagnosis.

Progression and management

The quoted median survival of 3 years may be much longer in patients who are asymptomatic at presentation. More recently, it has been shown that the presence of anaemia, a very high or low white cell count, the presence of bone marrow chromosomal abnormalities and advanced patient age are all associated with a worse prognosis, as is the presence of the JAK2 V617F mutation (Box 4.7).

Box 4.6 **Causes of a leucoerythroblastic blood film**

- Idiopathic myelofibrosis
- Bone marrow infiltration
- Severe sepsis
- Severe haemolysis
- Sick neonate
- Administration of haemopoietic growth factors
- Acute and chronic leukaemia (some types)

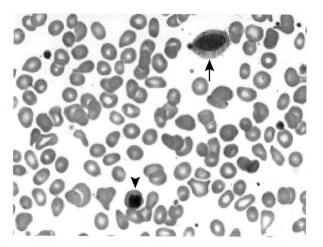

Figure 4.7 Leucoerythroblastic blood film in a patient with idiopathic myelofibrosis. Note the nucleated red blood cell (arrowhead) and the myelocyte (arrow).

Box 4.7 **Features of a poor prognosis in myelofibrosis**

- Haemoglobin < 10 g/dL
- White cell count < 4 or > 30×10^9/L
- Bone marrow chromosomal abnormalities
- Advanced patient age
- Raised number of CD34-positive cells in the peripheral blood
- Presence of JAK2 V617F mutation

Bone marrow transplantation from a matched sibling or unrelated donor should be offered to young patients with poor prognostic features. This is the only curative treatment modality for myelofibrosis, but, in view of its toxicity, it cannot be performed in the majority of patients with this disorder, who are > 50 years old at diagnosis.

Supportive blood transfusion may be needed for anaemic patients. Cytotoxic agents may be useful in the proliferative phase, particularly if the platelet count is raised. More recently, antifibrotic and antiangiogenic agents, such as thalidomide, have been used to inhibit progression of fibrosis, but success has been limited. Androgenic steroids, such as danazol and oxymethalone, can improve haemoglobin in a proportion of anaemic patients. There is also considerable interest in the possibility that it may be feasible to design specific inhibitors of activated (mutant) JAK2.

Splenectomy may improve the quality of life (although not the prognosis) by reducing the need for transfusions or the pain sometimes associated with a very enlarged spleen. Operative morbidity and mortality can be high, and are usually secondary to thrombosis or haemorrhage, making preoperative correction of coagulation abnormalities imperative. Low-dose irradiation of the spleen may be helpful in frail patients.

Death can be due to haemorrhage, infection or transformation to acute leukaemia. Portal hypertension with varices, iron overload from blood transfusion and compression of vital structures by extramedullary haemopoietic masses may also contribute to morbidity and mortality.

Further reading

Barosi G, Hoffman R. Idiopathic myelofibrosis. *Seminars in Hematology* 2005; **42**: 248–58.

Campbell PJ, Green AR. Management of polycythemia vera and essential thrombocythemia. *Hematology* 2005; 201–8.

Finazzi G, Harrison C. Essential thrombocythemia. *Seminars in Hematology* 2005; **42**: 230–8.

Tefferi A, Barbui T. BCR/ABL-negative, classic myeloproliferative disorders: diagnosis and treatment. *Mayo Clinic Proceedings* 2005; **80**: 1220–32.

Vassiliou GS, Green AR. Postgraduate haematology. Chapter 46. In: Hoffbrand AV, Catovsky D & Tuddenham EGD, eds. *The Myeloproliferative Disorders*. Blackwell Publishing, Oxford, 2006.

Acknowledgement

We thank Dr Ellie Nacheva for the fluorescence in situ hybridization image showing deletion of the long arm of chromosome 20.

CHAPTER 5

Chronic Myeloid Leukaemia

John M Goldman

OVERVIEW

- The presence of the *bcr-abl* fusion gene expressed as a p210Bcr-Abl oncoprotein is diagnostic of CML

- The *bcr-abl* gene is almost always localized to a 22q– (or Philadelphia) chromosome

- With tyrosine kinase inhibitors (TKIs e.g. imatinib) the duration of chronic phase disease is much longer than with earlier therapy

- TKIs are therefore the best initial therapy for CML

- Allografting is currently reserved for patients who fail TKIs

Chronic myeloid leukaemia (CML) is a clonal malignant myeloproliferative disorder believed to originate in a single abnormal haemopoietic stem cell. The progeny of this abnormal stem cell proliferate over months or years, so that, by the time the leukaemia is diagnosed, the bone marrow is grossly hypercellular and the number of leucocytes is greatly increased in the peripheral blood. Normal blood cell production is almost completely replaced by leukaemia cells, which, however, still function almost normally.

CML has an annual incidence of 1–1.5/100 000 of the population (in the UK about 700 new cases each year), with no clear geographical variation. Presentation may be at any age, but the peak incidence is at 50–70 years, with a slight male predominance. This leukaemia is very rare in children. Because the disease evolves very slowly and 'routine' blood counts are carried out increasingly frequently, today, up to 50% of patients are diagnosed before showing any symptoms.

Most cases of CML occur sporadically. The only known predisposing factor is irradiation as shown by studies of Japanese survivors of the atomic bombs and in patients who have received radiotherapy for ankylosing spondylitis and various neoplastic conditions.

The clinical course of CML can be divided into a chronic or 'stable' phase and an advanced phase, the latter term covering both accelerated and blastic phases. Most patients present with chronic phase disease, which in the past lasted on average 4–5 years. However, since the introduction into clinical practice of the new tyrosine kinase inhibitors (see p. 24), the median duration of the chronic phase may prove to be much longer, even 10–20 years. In about two-thirds of patients, the chronic phase transforms gradually into an accelerated phase, characterized by a moderate increase in blast cells, increasing anaemia or thrombocytosis, or other features not compatible with chronic phase disease. After a variable number of months, this accelerated phase progresses to frank acute blastic transformation. The remaining one-third of patients move abruptly from chronic phase to an acute blastic phase (or blastic crisis) without an intervening phase of acceleration.

Pathogenesis

All leukaemia cells in patients with CML contain a specific cytogenetic marker, described originally in 1960 by workers in Philadelphia, and thus known as the Philadelphia or Ph chromosome (Fig. 5.1). The Ph chromosome is derived from a normal 22 chromosome that has lost part of its long arm as a result of a balanced reciprocal translocation of chromosomal material involving one of each pair of chromosomes 9 and 22; thus the translocation is t(9;22)(q34;q11). The Ph chromosome (also known as 22q–) therefore appears somewhat shorter than its normal counterpart, and the 9q+ somewhat longer than the normal chromosome 9.

The Ph chromosome carries a specific fusion gene known as *bcr–abl*, which results from juxtaposition of part of the *abl* proto-oncogene (from chromosome 9) with part of the *bcr* gene on chromosome 22. This fusion gene is expressed as a specific messenger (m) RNA, which in turn generates a protein called p210Bcr–Abl. This protein perturbs stem cell kinetics and associated myelopoiesis, resulting in the chronic phase of CML, although the exact mechanism remains unclear.

The management of CML in the chronic phase was revolutionized in 1998 by the introduction of imatinib mesylate, which kills

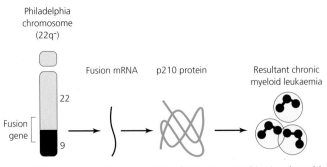

Figure 5.1 Formation of the Philadelphia chromosome resulting in a *bcr–abl* fusion gene that generates a fusion protein (p210) responsible for the chronic myeloid leukaemia (CML) phenotype.

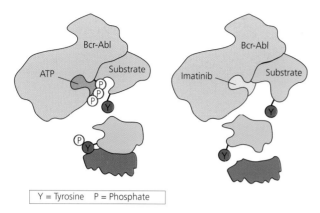

Figure 5.2 Mechanism of action of imatinib.

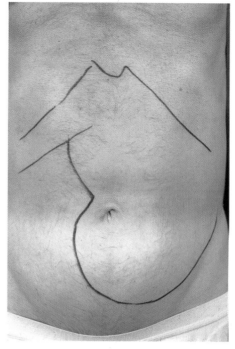

Figure 5.3 Patient with massive splenomegaly in chronic phase chronic myeloid leukaemia.

leukaemia cells by blocking the enzymatic function of the Bcr–Abl oncoprotein and thereby permits regeneration of normal haemopoietic cells (Fig. 5.2).

Chronic phase disease

Presentation

The characteristic symptoms of CML at presentation include fatigue, weight loss, sweating, anaemia, haemorrhage or purpura, and the sensation of a mass in the left upper abdominal quadrant (spleen) (Box 5.1). Often the disease is detected as a result of routine blood tests performed for unrelated reasons, and up to 50% of patients are totally asymptomatic at the time of diagnosis. The spleen may be greatly enlarged before the onset of symptoms. Treatment that reduces the leucocyte count to normal usually restores the spleen to normal size. Much rarer features at presentation include non-specific fever, lymphadenopathy, visual disturbances due to leucostasis (a form of hyperviscosity caused by an extremely high white cell count) or retinal haemorrhages, splenic pain due to infarction, gout and occasionally priapism.

The commonest physical sign at diagnosis is an enlarged spleen (Fig. 5.3), which may vary from being just palpable at the left costal margin to filling the whole left side of the abdomen and extending towards the right iliac fossa. The liver may be enlarged, with a soft, rather ill-defined lower edge. Spontaneous and excessive bruising in response to minor trauma is common.

Diagnosis

The diagnosis of CML in the chronic phase can be made from a study of the peripheral blood film (Fig. 5.4), which shows greatly increased numbers of leucocytes with many immature forms (promyelocytes and myelocytes) (Box 5.2); the marrow is usually examined to confirm the diagnosis (Box 5.3).

Marrow examination shows increased cellularity. The distribution of immature leucocytes resembles that seen in the blood film. Red cell production is relatively reduced. Megakaryocytes, the cells giv-

---

Box 5.1 **Clinical features in patients with CML at diagnosis**

Common
- Fatigue
- Weight loss
- Sweating
- Anaemia
- Haemorrhage: e.g. easy bruising, discrete ecchymoses
- Splenomegaly with or without hepatomegaly

Rare
- Splenic infarction
- Leucostasis
- Gout
- Retinal haemorrhages
- Priapism
- Fever

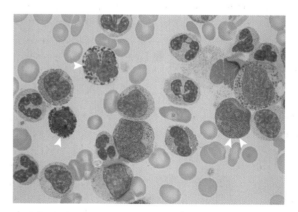

Figure 5.4 Peripheral blood film from a patient with chronic myeloid leukaemia showing many mature granulocytes, including two basophils (arrow); a blast cell is prominent (double arrow).

ing rise to platelets, are plentiful but may be smaller than usual and morphologically atypical.

Reverse transcriptase polymerase chain reaction (RT-PCR) confirms the presence of a *bcr–abl* fusion. Cytogenetic study of marrow shows the presence of the Ph chromosome in all dividing cells.

The patient's blood concentrations of urea and electrolytes are usually normal at diagnosis, whereas the lactate dehydrogenase is usually raised. Serum urate concentration may be raised (Fig. 5.5).

Management

After diagnosis, the first priority is a frank discussion with the patient. It is now customary to use the term leukaemia in this discussion and to explain to the patient that he or she may expect to live for many years with a normal lifestyle (Box 5.4). The clinician should explain the propensity of the disease to progress to an advanced phase. The options for initial treatment should be discussed, but in

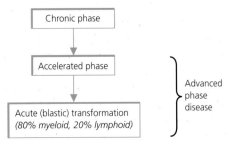

Figure 5.5 Course of chronic myeloid leukaemia, showing progression to blastic phase.

practice most patients are advised to start treatment with imatinib mesylate (Glivec ®; Novartis) or an imatinib-containing combination. Younger men should be offered cryopreservation of semen if necessary.

If CML is diagnosed in pregnancy, the woman should have the chance to continue to term. CML has no adverse effect on pregnancy and pregnancy has no adverse effect on CML.

The clinician may wish to mention at this point the existence of patient information booklets produced by the British Association of Cancer United Patients (BACUP) and by the Leukaemia Research Fund, which are extremely valuable, as many patients will not retain all that is said at this first interview. There are also a number of useful websites available on the Internet, although some of these are somewhat one-sided.

Imatinib mesylate

Imatinib is the treatment of choice for CML presenting in chronic phase. It acts by specifically inhibiting the enhanced protein tyrosine kinase activity of the Bcr–Abl oncoprotein and kills leukaemia cells by inducing apoptosis. The standard dose is 400 mg/day but it is possible that higher doses (i.e. 600 or 800 mg daily) may prove superior. It induces complete haematological remission in >95% of previously untreated patients and 70–80% of these will achieve complete cytogenetic remission. The best way of monitoring the patient's response to imatinib is by regular assay of Bcr–Abl transcript numbers in the peripheral blood using the real-time quantitative RT–PCR technology. Results are best expressed as a ratio of Bcr–Abl transcript numbers to a control transcript or as 'log reduction' from a baseline value. The rationale for regular monitoring is based on the observation that the degree to which the residual leukaemia is reduced predicts the duration of progression-free survival.

There are various possibilities for managing the patient who cannot tolerate or becomes resistant to imatinib but whose disease is still in the chronic phase. There is a good case for proceeding to allogeneic stem cell transplantation if the patient is relatively young (<55 years) and has an HLA (human leucocyte antigen) identical sibling or a well matched volunteer donor from the general population. A very reasonable alternative and the best option for the patient without any possible transplant donor would be to switch from imatinib to a second generation tyrosine kinase inhibitor, namely dasatinib (Sprycel, Bristol-Myers Squibb) or nilotinib (Tasigna, Novartis).

Dasatinib

This second generation tyrosine kinase inhibitor is active against both Abl and Src oncogenes and *in vitro* studies show it to be about 300 times more active than imatinib. It has demonstrated considerable efficacy in patients resistant to imatinib and patients who respond well should probably be continued on the drug indefinitely. The recommended dose is currently 100 mg daily.

Nilotinib

This agent, also a second generation tyrosine kinase inhibitor, is also active in patients whose leukemia appears resistant to imatinib. The currently recommended dose is 800 mg daily. At present there is no clear reason for preferring dasatinib to nilotinib or vice versa.

Hydroxyurea

Hydroxyurea is a ribonucleotide reductase inhibitor, which is remarkably effective at controlling symptoms and reducing the leucocyte count in chronic phase CML. It does not reduce the proportion of Ph-positive cells in the bone marrow and there is little evidence that it prolongs life to any extent. It is useful as a short-term measure for newly diagnosed patients or as an interim measure for patients resistant to imatinib while other more definitive treatments are being considered. The standard dose is 2.0 g daily. Toxicity includes rashes, gastrointestinal upset and mouth ulceration, but side effects are actually very rare at standard dosage.

Interferon-α

Interferon-α is a member of a family of naturally occurring glycoproteins with antiviral and antiproliferative actions. Side effects include short-term fever and flu-like symptoms and sometimes also persisting anorexia, weight loss, depression, alopecia, rashes, neuropathies, autoimmune disorders and thrombocytopenia. Currently, interferon-α should be considered for chronic phase patients resistant to imatinib mesylate.

Allogeneic stem cell transplantation

Patients younger than 60 years who prove resistant to imatinib at maximum dosage and who have siblings with identical HLA types

may be offered treatment by high-dose cytoreduction (chemotherapy and radiotherapy) followed by transplantation of haemopoietic stem cells collected from the donor's bone marrow or peripheral blood. With the typical family size in western Europe, about 30% of patients will have matched sibling donors. In selected cases, transplants may also be performed with HLA-identical unrelated donors. Allogeneic stem cell transplants are associated with an appreciable risk of morbidity and mortality, and, in general, older patients (40–60 years) fare less well than younger patients (Fig. 5.6). Nevertheless, the projected cure rate after allogeneic stem cell transplantation is about 60–70%.

Advanced phase disease

Presentation

Advanced phase disease may be diagnosed incidentally as a result of a blood test at a routine clinic visit. Alternatively, the patient may have excessive sweating, persistent fever, or otherwise unexplained symptoms of anaemia, splenic enlargement or infarction, haemorrhage, or bone pain. In most cases the blast crisis is myeloid (that is, resembling acute myeloid leukaemia), and in a fifth of cases lymphoid blast crisis occurs (Fig. 5.5).

Occasionally patients progress to a myelofibrotic phase of the disease, in which intense marrow fibrosis predominates, blast cells proliferate less aggressively, and the clinical picture is characterized by splenomegaly and pancytopenia consequent on marrow failure.

Management

Patients who present in accelerated phase may derive considerable short-term benefit from imatinib, which can re-establish chronic phase disease and even Ph-negative haemopoiesis in some cases. Conversely, imatinib has no role in the management of patients who received the drug for treatment of prior chronic phase disease. Such patients may still respond to hydroxyurea or busulfan if they have not previously received these agents. Splenectomy may be useful to improve thrombocytopenia or symptoms due to splenomegaly. Patients in a blastic phase respond only transiently to imatinib, although it may be reasonable to start their treatment with this agent at 800 mg/day. Thereafter, treatment should be continued within a few weeks by use of appropriate combination chemotherapy (see below), although the possibility of treating localized pain or resistant splenomegaly by radiotherapy should not be forgotten. For those patients with myeloid transformations, drugs suitable for treating acute myeloid leukaemia will control the leukaemic proliferation for a time. About 30% of patients will achieve a second chronic phase compatible with a normal lifestyle for months or years. Patients with lymphoid transformations should be treated with drugs appropriate to adult acute lymphoblastic leukaemia. Second chronic phase may be achieved in 40–60% of cases, more commonly in those who had a short interval from diagnosis to transformation. Patients restored to second chronic phase should receive prophylaxis against neuroleukaemia, comprising five or six intrathecal injections of methotrexate, but there is no indication for cranial or craniospinal irradiation.

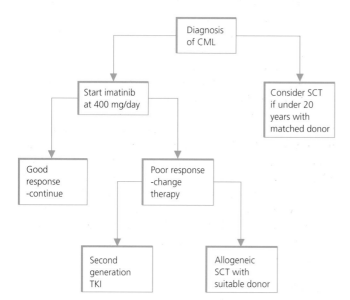

Figure 5.6 Possiblr scheme for managing patients presenting with CML in chronic phase. (See Baccarani, *et al.* 2006 for response criteria.)

Further reading

Baccarani M, Saglio G, Goldman JM *et al*. Evolving concepts in the management of chronic myeloid leukemia: recommendations from an expert panel on behalf of the European Leukemia-net. *Blood* 2006; **108**: 1809-20.

Deininger M, Goldman JM, Melo JM. The molecular biology of chronic myeloid leukemia. *Blood* 2000; **96**: 3343–56.

Druker BJ, Guilhot P, O'Brien SG *et al*. Five-year follow-up of imatinib therapy for newly diagnosed chronic-phase chronic myeloid leukemia. *New Eng J Med* 2006; **355**: 2408–17.

Goldman JM, Druker B. Chronic myeloid leukemia: current treatment options. *Blood* 2001; **98**: 2039–42.

Goldman JM, Melo JV. Chronic myeloid leukemia. *New England Journal of Medicine* 2003; **349**: 1449–62.

Hughes T, Deininger M, Hochhaus A *et al*. Monitoring CML patients responding to treatment with tyrosine kinase inhibitors – recommendations for 'harmonizing' current methodology for detecting BCR-ABL transcripts and kinase domain mutations and for expressing results. *Blood* 2006; **108**: 28-37.

Hughes TP, Kaeda J, Branford S *et al*. Frequency of major molecular responses to imatinib or interferon alfa plus cytarabine in newly diagnosed chronic myeloid leukemia. *New England Journal of Medicine* 2003; **349**: 1421–30.

O'Brien SG, Guilhot F, Larson RA *et al*. Interferon and low dose cytarabine compared with imatinib for newly diagnosed chronic phase chronic myeloid leukemia. *New England Journal of Medicine* 2003; **348**: 994–1004.

Sawyers C. Chronic myeloid leukemia. *New England Journal of Medicine* 1999; **340**: 1330–40.

CHAPTER 6

The Acute Leukaemias

Mark Cook, Charles Craddock

OVERVIEW

- Acute leukaemias develop as a consequence of acquired genetic abnormalities in haemopoietic stem cells
- Acute leukaemias can be subdivided into acute myeloid leukaemia (AML) and acute lymphoblastic leukaemia (ALL)
- AML and ALL both present with symptoms of bone marrow failure caused by anaemia, neutropenia or thrombocytopenia
- Chromosomal (cytogenetic) abnormalities define different biological subgroups of AML and ALL
- Patient age, cytogenetic classification and response to initial chemotherapy are important factors allowing risk stratification
- Treatment of both ALL and AML is initially with myelosuppressive chemotherapy
- Allogeneic stem cell transplantation is reserved for patients predicted to have a poor outcome with chemotherapy alone

Acute leukaemia is a malignant disorder of white cells caused by a failure of normal differentiation of haemopoietic stem cells and progenitors into mature cells. This results in the accumulation of primitive leukaemic cells within the bone marrow cavity, causing bone marrow failure, and as a consequence patients typically present with anaemia, thrombocytopenia or neutropenia (Box 6.1).

Much progress has been made in understanding the pathogenesis of the acute leukaemias, and it is now clear that they occur because of the acquisition of distinct genetic abnormalities in haemopoietic stem cells or committed progenitors. These molecular abnormalities frequently occur as the result of chromosomal translocations or the loss of chromosomal material. In addition, activating mutations in genes regulating cellular proliferation, such as tyrosine kinase genes, are commonly identified. Malignant transformation of primitive cells with the capacity to develop into cells of the myeloid lineage results in acute myeloid leukaemia (AML), while acquired genetic abnormalities in lymphoid progenitors result in acute lymphoblastic leukaemia (ALL).

In the past 30 years there has been a steady improvement in survival rates in patients presenting with acute leukaemia, most dramatically in childhood ALL. This progress has occurred as a result of the rigorous evaluation of chemotherapeutic drugs and supportive care in the setting of large-scale randomized studies. The recent identification of specific molecular abnormalities associated with the pathogenesis of acute leukaemia now also offers the prospect of designing new therapies that target the underlying molecular lesion.

Classification

The acute leukaemias are subdivided into (i) AML and (ii) ALL. AML is a disease of myeloid progenitors (cells from which neutrophils, eosinophils, monocytes, basophils, megakaryocytes and erythrocytes are derived) and is characterized by the accumulation of myeloblasts within the bone marrow (Fig. 6.1). ALL, in contrast, is a disease of lymphoid progenitors (immature lymphocytes) resulting in infiltration of the bone marrow by lymphoblasts (Fig. 6.2).

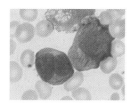

Figure 6.1 Myeloblasts and pathognomonic Auer rod in a patient with acute myeloid leukaemia.

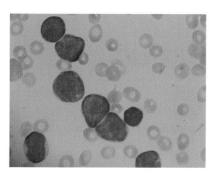

Figure 6.2 Lymphoblasts in a patient with acute lymphoblastic leukaemia.

Box 6.1 **Presenting symptoms in acute leukaemia**

- Symptoms of anaemia: fatigue, shortness of breath
- Complications of neutropenia: fever, cough, sore throat, cellulitis
- Complications of thrombocytopenia: petechiae, bleeding, bruising

For nearly three decades, the French–American–British (FAB) classification was used to subdivide AML and ALL based on morphological criteria. The recent identification of non-random cytogenetic abnormalities in AML has been incorporated into the new World Health Organization (WHO) classification, which includes karyotypic as well as morphological abnormalities (http://www3.who.int/icd/vol1htm2003/fr-icd.htm).

Epidemiology

ALL is the commonest cancer of childhood. The highest incidence is in the age range 0–4 years (5.2 cases per 100 000 per annum) falling to 1.9 cases per 100 000 per annum in the 10–14-year age group. After 40 years of age, there is a secondary rise in incidence but not to the levels seen in childhood. US data suggest that ALL is more common in white than in African American children. Conversely, AML is more common in adulthood, with an overall incidence of 3.4 per 100 000 per annum, and nearly two-thirds of cases occurring in patients over the age of 60 years.

Although the great majority of cases of acute leukaemia are sporadic, a number of factors associated with an increased risk of developing leukaemia have been identified (Box 6.2).

Clinical features of acute leukaemia

Acute leukaemia can present with a wide range of symptoms and signs reflecting infiltration of the bone marrow or other organs with leukaemic blasts or the systemic consequences of advanced malignancy. It should be considered in the differential diagnosis of a number of common clinical presentations (Box 6.3).

> **Box 6.2 Risk factors for the development of acute leukaemia**
>
> The majority of cases of leukaemia have no apparent risk factors
>
> **Hereditary**
> - Down's syndrome
> - Fanconi's anaemia
> - Bloom's syndrome
> - Klinefelter's syndrome
> - Wiskott–Aldrich syndrome
> - Ataxia telangiectasia
> - Osteogenesis imperfecta
> - Severe combined immunodeficiency
> - Neurofibromatosis type 1
> - Increased risk in siblings of affected child
>
> **Acquired**
> *Carcinogen exposure*
> - Benzene
> - Radiation
>
> *Prior haematological disorder*
> - Myelodysplastic syndrome
> - Myeloproliferative disease
> - Aplastic anaemia
> - Paroxysmal nocturnal haemoglobinuria

> **Box 6.3 Differential diagnosis of acute leukaemia**
>
> **High white count/ circulating blasts on peripheral blood film due to other process**
> - 'Leukaemoid reaction', e.g. as seen in severe infection
> - Marrow infiltration by other malignant disease
>
> **Lymphadenopathy**
> - Lymphoma
> - Non-haemopoietic malignancy
> - Viral infection (e.g. infectious mononucleosis, human immunodeficiency virus)
> - Other infections (e.g. tuberculosis)
> - Autoimmune disease
>
> **Hepatosplenomegaly**
> - Lymphoproliferative disease
> - Myeloproliferative disease
> - Storage disease
> - Autoimmune disease
> - Tropical disease
>
> **Myelodysplasia**
>
> **Lymphoblastic lymphoma**

Infection

Neutropenia (reduced neutrophil count) is common at diagnosis, and results in an increased risk of both bacterial and fungal infection. Bacterial infection in the throat, skin or perianal region is commonly seen and may be missed unless the relevant areas are carefully examined. Fungal infections most commonly present either as oral candidiasis or invasive intrapulmonary aspergillosis. Even if the neutrophil count appears normal, neutrophil function can often be poor, particularly in patients with a prior history of myelodysplastic syndrome in which neutrophils are usually dysfunctional.

Bleeding

Bleeding can occur as a consequence of thrombocytopenia or abnormal coagulation. Spontaneous bruising, gingival bleeding, palatal and retinal haemorrhages, epistaxis, menorrhagia and prolonged bleeding after venepuncture are all relatively common.

Infiltration

Leukaemic blasts can infiltrate any organ. Bone pain is a direct consequence of marrow disease. Infiltration of the meninges, resulting in headache or cranial nerve palsies, is particularly common in ALL and consequently lumbar puncture is mandatory in newly diagnosed patients with ALL. Hepatosplenomegaly is frequently present at diagnosis in ALL, and mediastinal enlargement is well documented in T-cell ALL. ALL can also involve the testes, presenting with a painful testicular mass. Skin and gum infiltration also occur: most commonly in AML.

Diagnosis of acute leukaemia

A diagnosis of acute leukaemia is confirmed by the demonstration of an infiltrate of leukaemic blasts in the bone marrow. In all patients in whom intensive treatment is planned, the following investigations are mandatory.

Full blood count

The blood count is nearly always abnormal in acute leukaemia. Patients with acute leukaemia commonly present with circulating leukaemic blasts in the peripheral blood resulting in a raised white blood count. This will usually be accompanied by thrombocytopenia, neutropenia and anaemia. In a proportion of patients, the white blood count will be normal or reduced.

Coagulation

Thrombocytopenia is a common cause of petechial bleeding or bruising. Disseminated intravascular coagulation (DIC) is often present in newly diagnosed patients with acute leukaemia and may result in life-threatening bleeding complications. DIC is either triggered directly by the underlying leukaemia [acute promyelocytic leukaemia (APL) is typically associated with DIC] or can be secondary to sepsis. Consequently, measurement of the platelet count, prothrombin time, activated partial thromboplastin time and fibrinogen and, if abnormal, prompt correction, is essential in all newly diagnosed patients.

Biochemistry

Abnormal renal function can occur secondary to hyperuricaemia (particularly in association with a high white blood cell count) and sepsis. Infiltration of the liver can cause abnormal liver function tests.

Bone marrow aspirate and trephine biopsy

A diagnosis of leukaemia can usually be made from a bone marrow aspirate alone. Slides from a bone marrow aspirate are air-dried and stained within the haematology laboratory, making it possible to confirm the diagnosis on the same day as the test is performed. In patients with a heavy infiltrate of leukaemic cells, a bone marrow aspirate may sometimes fail to yield sufficient marrow cells (a 'dry tap') or only result in a haemodilute sample. In such circumstances, a trephine biopsy is needed, which requires a number of days to process in the laboratory.

Immunophenotyping

Leukaemic blasts are characterized by the aberrant expression of haemopoietic antigens on their cell surface. Distinct patterns of antigen expression permit accurate discrimination between myeloblasts and lymphoblasts, allowing confident distinction between AML and ALL. Current guidelines for immunophenotyping are available online (http://www.blackwell-synergy.com/links/doi/10.1046/j.1365–2257.2002.00135.x/full/;jsessionid=aTVogw__Pie66BGY5K).

Cytogenetic and molecular studies

The demonstration that specific chromosomal abnormalities are associated with distinct subtypes of acute leukaemia has had enormous implications for the diagnosis and management of acute leukaemia and it is now clear that distinct cytogenetic abnormalities present in newly diagnosed patients with acute leukaemia provide vitally important prognostic information. In AML, cytogenetic examination

at diagnosis can be used to classify patients into three prognostic risk groups. Patients with the chromosomal abnormalities t(8;21) (Fig. 6.3), inv(16) or t(15;17) have a relatively good prognosis when treated with intensive chemotherapy, whereas patients with abnormalities of chromosomes 3, 5 or 7 or complex karyotypic abnormalities respond poorly to chemotherapy. In ALL, cytogenetics also provides important prognostic information with the presence of the Philadelphia chromosome [t(9;22)] predicting poor long-term disease-free survival, whereas hyperdiploid karyotypes are associated with an improved outcome.

Many of the common translocations present in AML or ALL result in the formation of a novel gene, which can be detected in the bone marrow by the polymerase chain reaction (PCR). This allows confirmation of diagnosis and permits the monitoring of the response to treatment. This is best illustrated by APL, a particular subtype of AML, which is associated with the presence of the t(15;17) translocation (Fig. 6.4), which results in the formation of a novel gene, *PML:RARA*. Detection of the t(15;17) translocation or the *PML:RARA* transcript by PCR can be used both to confirm a diagnosis of APL and to monitor for the presence of minimal residual disease (MRD). Several other non-random chromosomal abnormalities,

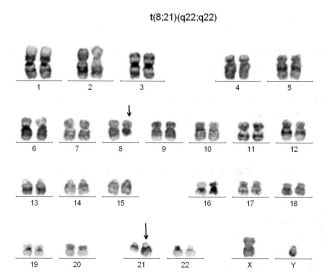

Figure 6.3 Karyotypic analysis in a patient with acute myeloid leukaemia associated with t(8;21).

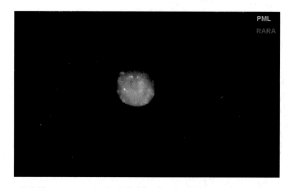

Figure 6.4 Fluorescence *in situ* hybridization study in a patient with acute promyelocytic leukaemia demonstrating t(15;17).

such as t(8;21) and inv(16), and their associated transcripts AML:ETO and CBFb:MYH11, are classically seen in AML and assist both in assigning patients with AML to a particular molecular subgroup and in monitoring MRD.

Chest radiography

A mediastinal mass may be present, particularly in T-cell ALL.

Lumbar puncture in patients with ALL

The presence of leukaemia in the central nervous system (CNS) should be suspected if there are symptoms of headache, visual disturbance or abnormalities such as blurred disc margins or retinal haemorrhage on fundoscopy. It is common at diagnosis and relapse in ALL but only rarely occurs in AML.

Principles of treatment

Acute leukaemia is a life-threatening, but potentially curable, disease and should be managed by a specialist multidisciplinary team. All patients in whom acute leukaemia is suspected or has been confirmed should be urgently referred to a specialist haematology unit. The essential early principles of management are summarized in Box 6.4. The most important prognostic factors in AML are patient age, performance status and presentation cytogenetics. It is important to assess whether patients have a significant chance of benefit from intensive chemotherapy. In patients whose outcome with chemotherapy is likely to be poor (such as patients over the age of 70 years with poor risk cytogenetics), palliative therapy with blood and platelet support may be the best treatment (Box 6.5 and Table 6.1). Such decisions are clearly complex and must be taken in careful consultation with the patients and their families.

Box 6.4 **Principles of management of acute leukaemia**

- Management in specialist unit by multidisciplinary team
- Prompt clinical assessment and, where appropriate, institution of supportive care
- Exclusion of significant coagulopathy
- Rapid diagnosis
- Discussion of diagnosis and treatment options with experienced clinician and clinical nurse specialist
- Rehydration and commencement of allopurinol (or, in patients at high risk of tumour lysis syndrome, rasburicase) in anticipation of treatment with chemotherapy
- Swift institution of intensive chemotherapy
- Institution of CNS-directed chemotherapy, where appropriate

---

Box 6.5 **Predictors of outcome in adults with acute leukaemia treated with intensive chemotherapy**

- Age
- Presenting white count
- Presentation cytogenetics
- Response to induction chemotherapy

Table 6.1 Predicted outcome in patients with acute leukaemia according to age and subtype

Type	Survival at 5 years
Childhood ALL	70–80%
Adult ALL	30–40%
Childhood AML	60%
AML (<55 years)	40%
AML (>55 years)	15%
AML >55 years with poor risk karyotype	<5%
APL	80%

ALL, acute lymphoblastic leukaemia; AML, acute myeloid leukaemia; APL, acute promyelocytic leukaemia.

Supportive care

Treatment and prevention of the complications caused by neutropenia and thrombocytopenia are vital both at diagnosis and during intensive treatment of acute leukaemia. This includes transfusion of platelet concentrates and prompt treatment of infection (Box 6.6). Careful examination and thorough investigation of neutropenic patients with a temperature >38°C is critical, since these patients are immunocompromised and susceptible to life-threatening infections. Particularly important sources of infection in neutropenic patients include bacterial and fungal pneumonias, infections associated with indwelling central lines and infections of the sinuses and perineum. Early institution of broad spectrum antibiotics after appropriate investigations (blood cultures, chest X-ray and swabs of potentially infected sites) is vital. If patients are hypotensive, aggressive treatment of possible septic shock including aggressive fluid resuscitation and, if necessary, transfer to the intensive care unit are critical.

General principles of management

The initial aim of treatment is to achieve a complete remission (CR), which is defined as the reduction of leukaemic blasts within the bone marrow to <5% and recovery of neutrophil and platelet counts. Once achieved, patients then receive further courses of chemotherapy with or without adjunctive stem cell transplantation with the aim of securing long-term disease erradication. The side effects of chemotherapy are varied (Box 6.7) but can be profound. It is most important to consider these when deciding whether to institute treat-

---

Box 6.6 **Supportive care**

- Inpatient care in a specialist unit
- Placement of long-term central venous catheter
- Red cell transfusion to maintain haemoglobin >8 g/dL
- Platelet transfusion to maintain platelet count >10 × 10⁹/L in patients unless patients are:
  - febrile
  - actively bleeding,
  in which case maintain platelet count >20 × 10⁹/L
- Institution of broad spectrum antibiotics in neutropenic patients with temperature >38.0°C

Box 6.7 **Side effects of chemotherapy**

Immediate
- Alopecia
- Nausea and vomiting
- Mucositis
- Hepatic dysfunction
- Haematological toxicity including neutropenia and thrombocytopenia
- Peripheral neuropathy (e.g. vincristine)
- Central nervous system toxicity (e.g. high-dose cytarabine)

Late
- Infertility
- Cardiomyopathy (e.g. anthracyclines)
- Pulmonary fibrosis
- Secondary malignancies including myelodysplasia and leukaemia
- Growth failure
- Cognitive dysfunction
- Pulmonary fibrosis

ment in older patients in whom the prospects for long-term survival with conventional chemotherapy are poor.

Specific management of AML

Chemotherapy

Effective chemotherapeutic agents in AML include the anthracyclines (daunorubicin and idarubicin), cytosine arabinoside and etoposide. A new drug currently being examined in the UK National Cancer Research Network (NCRN) AML studies is gemtuzumab ozogamicin, an immunoconjugate of the toxin calicheamycin and an antibody to CD33 – an antigen expressed on leukaemic cells. These drugs are administered in combination in order to increase their activity and reduce the risk of the emergence of drug resistance. CRs can be achieved in 70–80% of newly diagnosed adults using one or two cycles of induction chemotherapy. Once CR has been achieved, the majority of patients receive a further two cycles of chemotherapy. In APL, treatment with myelosuppressive drugs, particularly anthracyclines, is combined with all-*trans*-retinoic acid, which is very active in this disease and has substantially improved outcome.

Role of stem cell transplantation

Allogeneic stem cell transplantation using an HLA identical sibling has the capacity to reduce the relapse rate and improve disease-free survival in patients with AML. Allogeneic transplantation is not indicated in patients with good risk cytogenetics, whose outcome with chemotherapy alone is encouraging, but is an important treatment modality in patients under the age of 45 years with standard or poor risk cytogenetics in first CR.

One of the frustrations of stem cell transplantation has been the fact that the toxicity associated with conventional myeloablative conditioning regimens has precluded the use of this highly effective anti-leukaemia therapy in older patients. The recent demonstration that it is possible to significantly reduce the toxicity of allogeneic transplantation through the use of less intensive chemotherapy regi-

mens ('reduced intensity' or 'mini' transplants) has made it feasible to extend the curative potential of allogeneic stem cell transplantation to patients up to the age of 65 years – a remarkable breakthrough. Preliminary results using such reduced intensity transplants suggest that they may possess the capacity to improve the outcome of older patients with AML and this is currently being tested in national studies.

Management of relapse

Despite intensive treatment, leukaemic relapse occurs in the majority of adults with AML. Reinduction treatment and subsequent transplantation using a sibling or an unrelated donor represent the only curative treatment in the great majority of patients. The success of such an intensive treatment strategy is predictable at the time of relapse by three main factors: patient age, cytogenetics and duration of first remission. In patients whose duration of first remission is < 1 year, long-term survival rates even with intensive treatment are < 10%, and this information is clearly important when coming to a decision with the patient on whether to proceed down such an arduous road.

Novel therapies

There is clearly a need for the development of new treatments in AML. The success of imatinib (Glivec®; Novartis) in patients with chronic myeloid leukaemia (CML) has led to the hope that it may be possible to identify similar targets in AML. Although there has been some encouraging preliminary experience in AML with drugs which target dysregulated genes, such as *flt 3* or *ras*, in AML these agents have not as yet fulfilled their promise.

Specific management of ALL

Treatment of ALL follows the same principles as for AML with three main exceptions. Firstly, treatment directed at treating or preventing the seeding of the CNS with leukaemic blasts forms a central part of ALL regimens. Treatment takes three forms: (i) regular intrathecal administration of chemotherapy agents which are both active and non-toxic (such as methotrexate, cytosine arabinoside or steroids); (ii) the systemic administration of high-dose methotrexate; and (iii) cranial radiotherapy.

Secondly, several additional drugs including vincristine and L-asparaginase are highly active in ALL. In addition, imatinib is highly active in patients with Philadelphia-positive ALL and an important adjunct to conventional chemotherapy in this subgroup of usually adult patients.

Lastly, maintenance treatment for up to 2 years with oral drugs such as 6-mercaptopurine and methotrexate has been shown to improve overall survival in adults and children with ALL.

Allogeneic stem cell transplantation has an important role in the management of ALL. Although usually reserved for children and for patients who have previously relapsed, it plays an important role in preventing relapse and improving overall survival in adults with ALL in first CR. In adults lacking a sibling donor, unrelated donor transplantation is indicated, particularly in those deemed to be at high risk of relapse, such as patients with the Philadelphia chromosome.

Further reading

Burnett AK. Acute myeloid leukaemia: treatment of adults under 60 years. *Reviews in Clinical and Experimental Haematology* 2002; **6**: 26–45.

Grimwade D, Walker H, Oliver F *et al.* The importance of diagnostic cytogenetics on outcome in AML; analysis of 1612 patients entered into the MRC AML 10 trial. *Blood* 1998; **92**: 2322–33.

Lowenberg B, Downing JR, Burnett A. Acute myeloid leukemia. *New England Journal of Medicine* 1999; **341**: 1051–62.

Pui CH, Evans WE. Treatment of acute lymphoblastic leukemia. *New England Journal of Medicine* 2006; **12**: 166–78.

Tauro S, Craddock C, Peggs K *et al.* Allogeneic stem cell transplantation using a reduced intensity conditioning (RIC) regimen has the capacity to produce durable remissions and long term disease free survival in patients with high risk acute myeloid leukemia (AML) and myelodysplasia (MDS). *Journal of Clinical Oncology* 2005; **23**: 9387–93.

Acknowledgements

The authors acknowledge the generosity of Matt Lawes and Mike Griffiths in the provision of photomicrographs.

CHAPTER 7

Platelet Disorders

Marie A Scully, Samuel J Machin, R J Leisner

OVERVIEW

- Platelets are produced from bone marrow megakaryocytes
- They are important in the formation of platelet plugs during normal haemostasis
- Surface glycoprotein receptors on platelets are important in platelet–platelet and platelet–endothelial cell adhesion
- Release of platelet contents from storage organelles within platelets is important in platelet aggregation
- Surface phospholipid of platelets is important in interaction and activation of clotting factors in the coagulation pathway
- Congenital platelet disorders are divided into:
  - Platelet production, e.g. thrombocytopenia with absent radii syndrome, Wiskott–Aldrich syndrome
  - Functional platelet abnormalities, e.g. Bernard–Soulier syndrome, Glanzmann's thrombasthenia
- Acquired platelet abnormalities can be divided into:
  - Bone marrow failure, e.g. aplastic anaemia, leukaemic bone marrow infiltration
  - Peripheral consumption, e.g. idiopathic thrombocytopenic purpura, post-transfusion purpura, neonatal alloimmune thrombocytopenia, thrombotic thrombocytopenic purpura (TTP)
- A full bleeding history, drug history and review of the peripheral blood film are of primary importance in the differential diagnosis
- Increasingly, molecular diagnosis is useful in congenital abnormalities
- Available treatments depend on the diagnosis:
  - Platelet concentrates (contraindicated in TTP)
  - Intravenous immunoglobulin
  - Tranexamic acid
  - Desmopressin
  - Recombinant factor VIIa
  - Bone marrow transplantation

Platelets are small anucleate cells produced predominantly by the bone marrow megakaryocytes as a result of budding of the cytoplasmic membrane. Megakaryocytes are derived from the haemopoietic stem cell, which is stimulated to differentiate to mature megakaryocytes under the influence of various cytokines, including thrombopoietin. Platelets play a key role in securing primary haemostasis.

Once released from the bone marrow, young platelets are trapped in the spleen for up to 36 hours before entering the circulation, where they have a primary haemostatic role. Their normal lifespan is 7–10 days and the normal platelet count for all age groups is 150–450 $\times 10^9$/L. The mean platelet diameter is 1–2 μm, and the normal range for cell volume (mean platelet volume; MPV) is 8–11 fL. Although platelets are non-nucleated cells, those that have recently been released from the bone marrow contain RNA and are known as reticulated platelets. They normally represent 8–16% of the total count and they indirectly indicate the state of marrow production.

Normal haemostasis

The platelet membrane contains integral glycoproteins essential in the initial events of adhesion and aggregation, leading to the formation of the platelet plug during haemostasis (Fig. 7.1).

Glycoprotein receptors react with aggregating agents, such as collagen on the damaged vascular endothelial surface and fibrinogen and von Willebrand factor (VWF), to facilitate platelet–platelet and platelet–endothelial cell adhesion. The major glycoproteins are the Ib/IX complex, the main binding protein of which is VWF, and IIb/IIIa, which specifically binds fibrinogen. Storage organelles within the platelet include the 'dense' granules, which contain nucleotides,

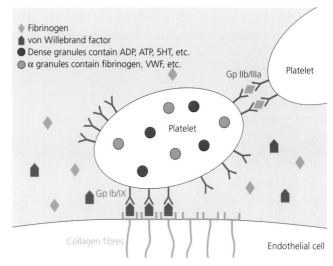

Figure 7.1 Normal platelet function.

calcium and serotonin, and α granules containing fibrinogen, VWF, platelet-derived growth factor and many other clotting factors. Following adhesion, the platelets are stimulated to release the contents of their granules, essential for platelet aggregation. The platelets also provide an extensive phospholipid surface for the interaction and activation of clotting factors in the coagulation pathway.

Congenital abnormalities

Congenital abnormalities of platelets can be divided into disorders of platelet production and those of platelet function. All are very rare. In general, they cause moderate to severe bleeding problems. Increasingly, the molecular basis for these disorders has been characterized and therefore can be used as a diagnostic tool, and may facilitate antenatal diagnosis.

Fanconi's anaemia

Fanconi's anaemia is an autosomal recessive preleukaemic condition, which often presents as thrombocytopenia with skeletal or genitourinary abnormalities. The cardinal laboratory feature is abnormal chromosomal fragility. The condition can be cured with bone marrow transplantation (BMT).

Thrombocytopenia with absent radii

Thrombocytopenia with absent radii (TAR) syndrome presents with the pathognomonic sign of bilateral absent radii (Fig. 7.2) and with severe (< 10 × 109/L) neonatal thrombocytopenia, although this often improves after the first year of life. This should be distinguished

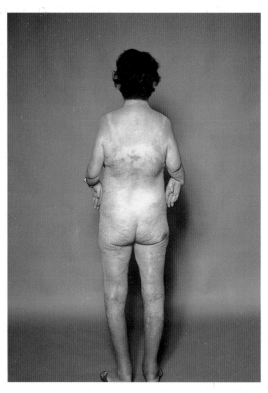

Figure 7.2 Amegakaryocytic thrombocytopenia with absent radii (TAR syndrome).

from amegakaryocytic thrombocytopenia, another leukaemia predisposition syndrome, in which severe neonatal thrombocytopenia is present with orthopaedic or neurological abnormalities in 10–30% of children. The underlying genetic abnormality, located to the c-mpl gene on chromosome 1, affects the thrombopoietin receptor.

Wiskott–Aldrich syndrome

This is an X-linked disorder with a triad of thrombocytopenia, eczema and T-cell immunodeficiency. The platelet count is usually 20–100 × 10⁹/L, and the platelets are small and functionally abnormal. The diagnosis can be confirmed by analysis of the *WAS* gene (Xp11). Like Fanconi's anaemia, this condition can only be cured with BMT.

MYH9-related thrombocytopenias

MYH9-related thrombocytopenias, including the May Hegglin anomaly, are autosomal dominant conditions associated with macrothrombocytopenia. The genetic abnormality is in the MYH9 gene, located on chromosome 22. Variants of Alport's syndrome are also characterized by giant platelets, associated with progressive hereditary nephritis and deafness (Fig. 7.3).

Disorders of the surface membrane

Disorders of the surface membrane are characterized by absence or abnormalities of platelet membrane glycoproteins, resulting in defective platelet adhesion and aggregation. These disorders include Bernard–Soulier syndrome, an autosomal recessive condition, and macrothrombocytopenia, a lack of VWF-dependent platelet agglutination, linked to genetic lesions of the glycoprotein (Gp)Ib/IX/V complex. Glanzmann's thrombasthenia is associated with abnormalities of the GpIIb/IIIa complex. In platelet-type von Willebrand's disease, spontaneous binding of plasma VWF to enlarged platelets results from mutations of GpIbα (Fig. 7.4).

Platelet storage pool diseases

Deficiencies in either the α or dense granules cause poor secondary platelet aggregation. Absence of α granules in Grey Platelet Syndrome, an autosomal dominant inherited condition, results in large, pale platelets on blood films.

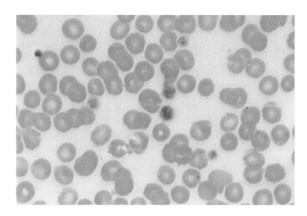

Figure 7.3 Giant granular platelets in peripheral blood film as seen in Bernard-Soulier syndrome or May Hegglin anomaly.

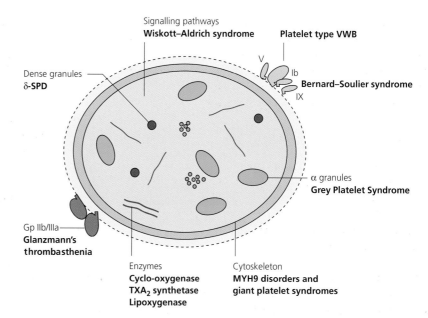

Figure 7.4 Site of abnormality in congenital platelet disorders.

Other conditions

There are also a variety of further specific surface membrane defects and internal enzyme abnormalities, which, although difficult to define, can cause troublesome chronic bleeding problems (Fig. 7.5).

Acquired abnormalities

Decreased production of platelets

Decreased platelet production caused by suppression or failure of the bone marrow is the commonest cause of thrombocytopenia. In aplastic anaemia, leukaemia and marrow infiltration, and after chemotherapy, thrombocytopenia is usually associated with a failure of red and white cell production, but may be an isolated finding secondary to drug toxicity (penicillamine, cotrimoxazole), alcohol, or viral infection (human immunodeficiency virus, infectious mononucleosis). Viral infection is the most common cause of mild transient thrombocytopenia (Box 7.1).

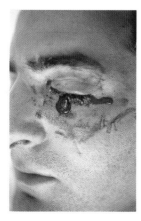

Figure 7.5 Bleeding around the eye in a patient with Bernard-Soulier syndrome.

Increased consumption of platelets

Increased platelet consumption may be due to immune or non-immune mechanisms.

Idiopathic thrombocytopenic purpura

Idiopathic thrombocytopenic purpura is a relatively common disorder and is the most frequent cause of an isolated thrombocytopenia without anaemia or neutropenia. In adults, it often presents insidiously, most frequently in women aged 15–50 years, and can be associated with other autoimmune diseases, in particular systemic lupus erythematosus or the primary antiphospholipid syndrome. In children, the onset is more acute and often follows a viral infection. The autoantibody produced is usually IgG, directed against antigens on the platelet membrane. Antibody-coated platelets are removed by the reticuloendothelial system, reducing the lifespan of the platelets to a few hours. The platelet count can vary from $<5 \times 10^9/L$ to near normal. The severity of bleeding is less than that seen with comparable degrees of thrombocytopenia in bone marrow failure, owing to the predominance of young, larger and functionally superior platelets (Figs 7.6 and 7.7, Box 7.2).

> **Box 7.1 Acquired disorders of reduced platelet production due to bone marrow failure/replacement**
>
> - Drug-induced
> - Leukaemia
> - Metastatic tumour
> - Aplastic anaemia
> - Myelodysplasia
> - Cytotoxic drugs
> - Radiotherapy
> - Associated with infection
> - Megaloblastic anaemia

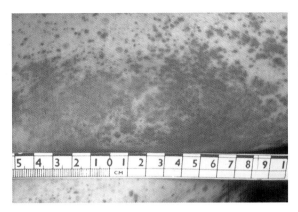

Figure 7.6 Spontaneous skin purpura in severe autoimmune thrombocytopenia.

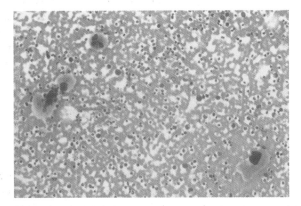

Figure 7.7 Bone marrow aspirate showing increased megakaryocytes in immune thrombocytopenia.

Box 7.2 Disorders with increased consumption of platelets

- Disorders with immune mechanism
  - Autoimmune: idiopathic thrombocytopenic purpura
  - Alloimmune: post-transfusion purpura, neonatal alloimmune thrombocytopenia
- Infection-associated: infectious mononucleosis, HIV, malaria
- Drug-induced: heparin, penicillin, quinine, sulphonamides, rifampicin
- Thrombotic thrombocytopenic purpura/haemolytic uraemic syndrome
- Hypersplenism and splenomegaly
- Disseminated intravascular coagulation
- Massive transfusion

Post-transfusion purpura

Post-transfuson purpura is a rare complication of blood transfusion. It presents with severe thrombocytopenia 7–10 days after the transfusion and usually occurs in multiparous women who are negative for the human platelet antigen (HPA)1a. Antibodies to HPA1a develop and, in some way, this alloantibody is responsible for the immune destruction of autologous (patient's own) platelets.

Neonatal alloimmune thrombocytopenia

Neonatal alloimmune thrombocytopenia is similar to haemolytic disease of the newborn except that the antigenic stimulus comes from platelet specific antigens rather than red cell antigens. In 80% of cases, the antigen is HPA1a and mothers who are negative for this antigen (about 5% of the population) form antibodies when sensitized by a fetus positive for the antigen. Fetal platelet destruction results from transplacental passage of these antibodies, and severe bleeding, including intracranial haemorrhage, can occur *in utero*. Firstborns are frequently affected and successive pregnancies are equally or more affected.

Heparin-induced thrombocytopenia

Heparin-induced thrombocytopenia occurs during unfractionated heparin therapy in up to 5% of patients, but is less frequently associated with low molecular weight heparins. It may become manifest when arterial or venous thrombosis occurs during a fall in the platelet count and is thought to be due to the formation of antibodies to heparin that are bound to platelet factor 4, a platelet granule protein. The immune complexes activate platelets and endothelial cells, resulting in thrombocytopenia. Heparin-induced thrombocytopenia carries an appreciable morbidity and mortality, especially from resulting thrombosis, if the diagnosis is delayed.

Thrombotic thrombocytopenic purpura

The hallmarks of thrombotic thrombocytopenic purpura are thrombocytopenia and microangiopathic haemolytic anaemia with clinical symptoms affecting any organ, but primarily manifesting as neurological symptoms, resulting from microvascular thrombosis. The condition is associated with deficiency of ADAMTS 13, a metalloprotease enzyme responsible for cleaving the ultra-high molecular weight multimers of VWF. The condition is suspected clinically by thrombocytopenia, red cell fragmentation on the blood film and a reticulocytosis. The demonstration of an abnormal pattern of von Willebrand multimers makes the diagnosis highly likely and the complete absence of the cleaving protease caused by an inhibitory antibody can be proven in some specialized laboratories (Fig. 7.8).

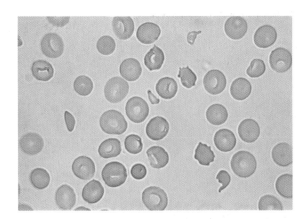

Figure 7.8 Red cell fragmentation in patient who presented with confusion and lethargy in whom thrombotic thrombocytopenic purpura was diagnosed. She responded well to large volume plasma exchange for one week.

Microangiopathic thrombocytopenia

Microangiopathic thrombocytopenia includes disorders such as pre-eclampsia or HELLP (*h*aemolysis, *e*levated *l*iver enzymes, *l*ow *p*latelets) syndrome in pregnancy, haemolytic uraemic syndrome, disseminated intravascular coagulation (DIC) and catastrophic antiphospholipid syndrome. The blood films may be similar in all these disorders, with thrombocytopenia, anaemia and fragmented red blood cells.

Disseminated intravascular coagulation

DIC usually occurs in critically ill patients as a result of catastrophic activation of the coagulation pathway, often due to sepsis. Widespread platelet consumption occurs, causing thrombocytopenia.

Massive blood transfusion

In patients with life-threatening bleeding, transfusion of 8–10 units of red blood cells without replacing clotting factors or platelets may result in prolonged clotting screen and thrombocytopenia.

Massive splenomegaly

The spleen normally pools about a third of the platelet mass, but in massive splenomegaly this can increase up to 90%, resulting in apparent thrombocytopenia.

Drugs

Aspirin, non-steroidal anti-inflammatory agents and glycoprotein IIb/IIIa antagonists are the most common causes of acquired platelet dysfunction (Box 7.3). For this reason, aspirin and the IIb/IIIa antagonists are used therapeutically as antiplatelet agents. Aspirin acts by irreversibly inhibiting cyclo-oxygenase activity in the platelet, resulting in impairment of the granule release reaction and defective aggregation. The effects of a single dose of aspirin last for the lifetime of the platelet (7–10 days). Recently, clopidogrel, a thienopyridine derivative, has been introduced as an oral antiplatelet agent that inhibits adenosine diphosphate binding to the platelet membrane and is useful in patients who are intolerant or resistant to aspirin. It is becoming widely used as a prophylactic agent for myocardial ischaemia and related coronary syndromes.

Bleeding in uraemic patients

Bleeding most commonly results from defects in platelet adhesion or aggregation, although thrombocytopenia, severe anaemia with packed cell volume < 20% or coagulation defects can also contribute.

Box 7.3 **Causes of acquired platelet dysfunction**

- Aspirin and non-steroidal anti-inflammatory agents
- Penicillins and cephalosporins
- Uraemia
- Ethanol
- Liver disease
- Myeloproliferative disorders
- Myeloma
- Cardiopulmonary bypass
- Fish oils

Box 7.4 **Thrombocytosis**

- Essential (primary) thrombocytosis
- Reactive (secondary) thrombocytosis
- Infection
- Malignant disease
- Acute and chronic inflammatory diseases
- Pregnancy
- Postsplenectomy
- Iron deficiency
- Haemorrhage

Essential (primary) thrombocytosis and reactive (secondary) thrombocytosis

In these conditions, the platelet count is raised above the upper limit of normal. A wide range of disorders can cause a raised platelet count ($> 800 \times 10^9$/L) but patients are normally asymptomatic, except in essential thrombocytosis, when excessive spontaneous bleeding may develop when the count exceeds 1000×10^9/L. Antiplatelet drugs can be useful to prevent thrombosis in high risk patients, for example, postoperatively. Some myelodysplastic syndromes may be complicated by an acquired storage pool-type platelet disorder (Box 7.4).

History and examination of patients

Abnormal bleeding associated with thrombocytopenia or abnormal platelet function is characterized by spontaneous skin purpura and ecchymoses, mucous membrane bleeding and protracted bleeding after trauma. Prolonged nosebleeds can occur, particularly in children, and menorrhagia or postpartum haemorrhage is common in women. Rarely, subconjunctival, retinal, gastrointestinal, genitourinary and intracranial bleeds may occur. In thrombocytopenic patients, severe spontaneous bleeding is unusual with a platelet count $\geq 20 \times 10^9$/L, unless there is associated platelet dysfunction.

Investigations

The investigations in a suspected platelet disorder will depend on the presentation and history in each patient. If the bleeding is severe, the patient may need urgent hospital referral for prompt evaluation, diagnosis and treatment, which may entail blood product support. All patients should have a full blood count, coagulation and biochemical screen, and then further investigations depending on the results of these. A thorough review of the blood film can help in the diagnosis or exclusion of many disorders associated with thrombocytopenia (Fig. 7.9).

Thrombocytopenia can be artefactual and due to platelet clumping or a blood clot in the sample, which should be excluded in all cases. The skin bleeding time, which is invasive, variable and not reliable in screening mild platelet disorders, has been replaced by devices that perform an *in vitro* bleeding time on small volumes of citrated blood and simulate platelet function in a high shear rate situation. The sensitivity of these devices for all platelet disorders is still under investigation.

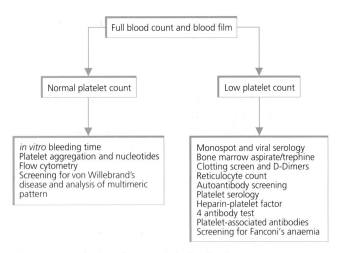

Figure 7.9 Investigation of suspected platelet disorder.

Management

All serious bleeding due to a platelet disorder needs haematological assessment and treatment. Mild or trivial bleeding due to a transient postviral thrombocytopenia or aspirin ingestion needs no active treatment and can be managed on an outpatient basis (Box 7.5).

Congenital disorders

A neonate or small infant with bleeding must be referred for evaluation as the inherited bleeding disorders (e.g. haemophilia or von Willebrand's disease) and platelet disorders can present at a very young age.

Severe bleeding episodes in all the congenital thrombocytopenias and platelet function disorders require filtered human leucocyte antigen-compatible platelet transfusions to secure haemostasis, although, in minor episodes in the dysfunctional syndromes, desmopressin (1-deamino-8-D-arginine vasopressin; DDAVP) given intravenously or intranasally with antifibrinolytics (tranexamic acid) may be sufficient. There is increasing evidence that, in selected patients with congenital disorders, recombinant factor VIIa (Novoseven®; Novartis) may be of use in the treatment or prevention of bleeding. It is licensed for use in patients with Glanzmann's thrombasthenia who have antibodies to the missing glycoprotein. This avoids exposure to blood products, but is expensive and the response may be variable. Bone marrow transplantation can potentially offer a cure in a number of these conditions.

Acquired disorders

In thrombocytopenia due to bone marrow failure or marrow infiltration, for example leukaemia or cancer, prophylactic platelet transfusions are given to keep the platelet count above 10×10^9/L, although the threshold is higher in infected or bleeding patients or to cover invasive procedures.

In childhood idiopathic thrombocytopenic purpura, spontaneous recovery is common, and treatment, such as corticosteroids, intravenous immunoglobulin or anti-D immunoglobulin, is given only in life-threatening bleeding. In adults, the condition rarely remits without treatment and is more likely to become chronic. Initial treatment is prednisolone 1mg/kg daily (80% of cases remit) and/

Box 7.5 Treatment of platelet disorders

Congenital disorders
- Platelet transfusions (leucodepleted, HLA compatible and irradiated)
- Desmopressin
- Tranexamic acid
- Recombinant factor VIIa
- Bone marrow transplantation

Acquired disorders
Bone marrow failure
- Platelet transfusions if platelet count < 10×10^9/L

Idiopathic thrombocytopenic purpura (adults)
- Prednisolone
- Intravenous immunoglobulin
- Anti-D immunoglobulin
- Rituximab
- Splenectomy

Post-transfusion purpura
- Intravenous immunoglobulin
- Plasma exchange

Heparin-induced thrombocytopenia
- Anticoagulation but without heparin
- Avoid platelet transfusions

Thrombotic thrombocytopenic purpura
- Large volume plasma exchange
- Aspirin when platelets > 50×10^9/L
- Avoid platelet transfusions

Disseminated intravascular coagulation
- Treat underlying cause
- Fresh frozen plasma
- Platelet transfusion

Hypersplenism
- Splenectomy if severe

Platelet function disorders
- Platelet transfusion
- Desmopressin (occasionally of use, e.g. in uraemia)
- Tranexamic acid

or intravenous immunoglobulin (0.4 g/kg for 5 days or 1 g/kg for 2 days), or both. More recently, the use of anti-D in Rh(D) positive patients has been associated with a 75% response rate. In refractory patients, splenectomy has a 60–70% chance of long-term cure, although the use of rituximab, an anti-CD20 monoclonal antibody, has proven equally effective, without the need for surgical intervention. Other potential therapies including azathioprine, danazol, vinca alkaloids and high-dose dexamethasone have all been tried with variable success.

Post-transfusion purpura may respond to intravenous immunoglobulin (at the doses given above), or plasma exchange may be required. Platelet transfusions should be avoided.

Patients in whom heparin-induced thrombocytopenia is suspected are often inpatients with ongoing thrombosis and may have complex medical problems. It is essential to stop heparin and treat thrombosis with other anticoagulants; further use of heparins should be avoided. Warfarin, synthetic heparinoids or ancrod can be used. Platelet transfusions are contraindicated in heparin-induced thrombocytopenia and in thrombotic thrombocytopenic purpura. If the latter is suspected clinically and on the basis of laboratory tests, large volume plasma exchange should be started immediately and continued daily until substantial clinical improvement occurs and all the results of haematological tests have normalized. Aspirin can be started once the platelet count is $> 50 \times 10^9$/L.

With DIC, it is essential to treat the underlying cause in addition to aggressive replacement of depleted clotting factors and platelets with blood products. In patients requiring massive blood transfusion, replacement with fresh frozen plasma (15 mL/kg) and a pool of platelets should be given with every 8–10 units of red cells received.

In pronounced bleeding or risk of bleeding due to the acquired disorders of platelet function, platelets usually have to be transfused to provide normally functioning platelets, although desmopressin and tranexamic acid can also be of value. Usually treatment may only be necessary to cover surgical procedures or major haemorrhage.

Further reading

Coller BS. Anti-GPIIb/IIIa drugs: current strategies and future directions. *Thrombosis and Haemostasis* 2001; **86**: 427–43.

Hardisty RM. Platelet functional disorders. Chapter 24. In: Lilleyman J, Hann I & Blanchette V, eds. *Pediatric Hematology*, 2nd edn. Churchill Livingstone, London, 2000.

Nurden AT. Qualitative disorders of platelets and megakaryocytes. *Journal of Thrombosis and Haemostasis* 2005; **3**: 1773–82.

Rendu F, Brohard-Bohn B. The platelet release reaction: granules' constituents, secretion and functions. *Platelets* 2001; **12**: 261–73.

Shapiro AP. Platelet function disorders. *Haemophilia* 2000; **6**: 120–7.

Siddiqui MAA Scott LJ. Recombinant factor VIIa (Eptacog alfa). A review of its use in congenital or acquired haemophilia and other congenital bleeding disorders. *Drugs* 2005; **65**: 1161–77.

Smith OP. Inherited and congenital thrombocytopenia. Chapter 21. In: Lilleyman J, Hann I & Blanchette V, eds. *Pediatric Hematology*, 2nd edn. Churchill Livingstone, London, 2000.

CHAPTER 8

The Myelodysplastic Syndromes

Paul A Cahalin, John A Liu Yin

OVERVIEW

- Myelodysplasia results in cytopenias, especially anaemia, with an increased risk of transformation to acute myeloid leukaemia
- It is a disease particularly affecting the elderly
- Prognosis is related to the cytogenetics of the malignant clone, the percentage of bone marrow blasts and the number of cytopenias
- Treatment ranges from supportive care with blood products, immunotherapy and chemotherapy to allogeneic bone marrow transplantation, depending on the age and fitness of the patient, and the severity of the myelodysplasia
- New promising agents, including lenalidomide and azacytidine, are currently undergoing clinical trials

Introduction

- The myelodysplastic syndromes (MDS) are a group of clonal haemopoietic disorders. They are characterized by:
  - Ineffective haemopoiesis resulting in peripheral blood cytopenias of all three lineages, but especially anaemia
  - Increased risk (30%) of transformation to acute myeloid leukaemia
- MDS is mainly a disease of the elderly, with a median age at diagnosis of 60–75 years. It does, however, affect younger adults also. MDS is rare in children, and is associated with genetic disorders such as Fanconi's anaemia.

Aetiology and pathogenesis

The myelodysplastic syndromes (MDS) are classified into two major groups, primary (or *de novo*) and secondary. Primary refers to the majority of cases, where the cause is unknown.

Secondary cases, when there is an identifiable cause for its development, comprise 10–20% of all MDS. There is a recognized association between exposure to occupational chemicals, especially benzene, and the subsequent development of MDS. More frequently, previous chemotherapy or radiotherapy may lead to MDS, and this is termed therapy-related MDS. High-dose chemotherapy before autologous bone marrow or peripheral blood stem cell transplantation, along with radiotherapy, is associated with the development of MDS, usu-

ally 4–7 years later. Exposure to alkylating agents, such as melphalan and cyclophosphamide, is also linked to subsequent MDS.

Compared to primary cases, therapy-related MDS is characterized by

- more severe cytopenias
- occurrence at a younger age
- a higher rate of transformation to acute leukaemia
- more clonal chromosomal abnormalities
- a generally poorer prognosis.

The initial steps in the pathogenesis of MDS involve DNA damage to a pluripotent stem cell. This leads to the development of a myelodysplastic clone, which has a growth advantage over other haemopoietic cells. There is increased cellular proliferation within the bone marrow, resulting in a hypercellular marrow. However, these cells do not differentiate properly and there is an increased rate of apoptosis (programmed cell death). This means that, despite the hypercellular marrow, fewer mature cells exit the marrow into the peripheral blood, resulting in peripheral blood cytopenias. T-cell-mediated destruction of marrow elements results in a hypocellular marrow in the minority of cases.

Recently, much attention has focused on the extra addition of methyl groups to many genes involved in cell cycle regulation. It appears that hypermethylation of many genes results in their silencing, particularly tumour suppressor genes, contributing to uncontrolled proliferation of the abnormal clone (Fig. 8.1).

Diagnosis

The diagnosis should be suspected in an elderly person with unexplained anaemia, usually macrocytic, with normal haematinic levels. It should also be suspected in cases of anaemia with involvement of the other lineages, namely thrombocytopenia and neutropenia. Referral to a haematologist is indicated if MDS is suspected. It is important to assess the patient when he or she is otherwise well, as acute illnesses may give an erroneous impression of bone marrow function.

Symptoms

Many patients may be asymptomatic and have a full blood count performed for incidental reasons. Other patients may have symptoms of bone marrow failure. These include symptoms from anaemia (shortness of breath, chest pain, fatigue), from thrombocytopenia (bruising,

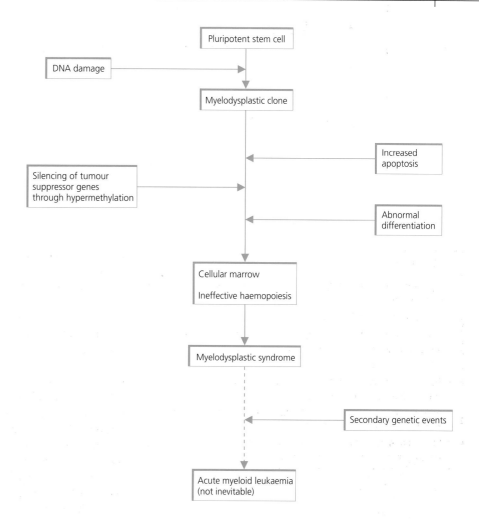

Figure 8.1 Pathogenesis of myelodysplastic syndromes.

bleeding) or from neutropenia (infections). Physical findings are often minimal, but may include pallor, purpura and rarely splenomegaly.

Investigations

The blood count and the blood film are vital in the diagnosis of MDS. It is very important to diagnose and correct B_{12} or folate deficiency before considering the diagnosis of MDS. Dysplastic features found in the peripheral blood and bone marrow are summarized in Table 8.1, although this list is not exhaustive.

However, to diagnose MDS confidently, a bone marrow aspirate and trephine biopsy are necessary. Many patients with suspected myelodysplasia will be very elderly with significant comorbidities, and may not require intervention, and therefore an invasive proce-

Table 8.1 Some changes that may be encountered in the peripheral blood and bone marrow in myelodysplastic syndromes

Red cells	White cells	Platelets
Peripheral blood		
Macrocytosis	Pseudo-Pelger neutrophils (Fig. 8.2)	Hypogranular
Anisocytosis (abnormal size)	Hypogranularity	
Poikilocytosis (abnormal shape)	Unusual nuclear shape	
Basophilic stippling		
Bone marrow		
Ringed sideroblasts (Fig. 8.3)	Pseudo-Pelger neutrophils	Micro-megakaryocytes
Binucleate or multinucleate precursors	Increased blasts	Megakaryocytes with separated nuclei (Fig. 8.4)

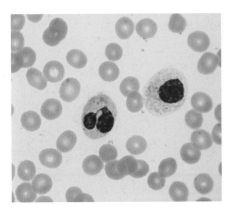

Figure 8.2 Pseudo-Pelger neutrophil (left) with a dysplastic neutrophil (right).

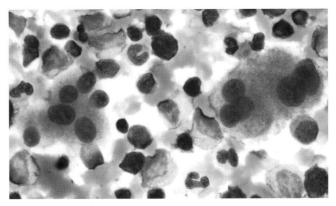

Figure 8.4 Dysplastic megakaryocytes with separated nuclei.

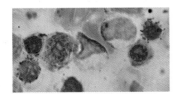

Figure 8.3 Ringed sideroblasts.

dure may not be necessary. However, all patients requiring regular therapy, including transfusion, should have the diagnosis confirmed with a bone marrow examination. It should be noted that dysplasia is not specific to MDS, and may be seen in other disorders, such as alcohol excess and cytotoxic therapy. It has therefore been suggested that at least 10% of the cells in a lineage should be dysplastic before that lineage is considered to be dysplastic.

Cytogenetics also gives important information. The presence of the same cytogenetic abnormality in multiple cells in the marrow gives more weight to the notion that the abnormality has arisen from a clonal disorder such as myelodysplasia. Cytogenetics is also very important in risk stratification, which has important implications on prognosis (see below). Notably, loss of the long arm of chromosome 5 (5q−) is found typically in middle aged women, and is associated with a long survival and a low risk of transformation to acute myeloid leukaemia (AML). Tissue typing is needed if stem cell transplantation is considered, especially in younger patients.

Classification

The classification of MDS was dominated until recently by the French–American–British (FAB) classification, proposed in 1982. However, more recently, the World Health Organization (WHO) has formulated a new classification (Table 8.2). Both classifications are based on the combination of peripheral blood and bone marrow

Table 8.2 Comparison of the French–American–British (FAB) and World Health Organization (WHO) classifications of myelodysplastic syndromes, with median survival times

FAB classification	WHO classification	Median survival in months (WHO types)
Refractory anaemia (RA)	Subdivided into:	
	RA	69
	Refractory cytopenias with multilineage dysplasia (RCMD)	33
Refractory anaemia with ringed sideroblasts (RARS)	Subdivided into:	
	RARS	69
	Refractory cytopenias with multilineage dysplasia and ringed sideroblasts (RCMD-RS)	32
Refractory anaemia with excess blasts (RAEB)	Subdivided into:	
	RAEB-1 (5–9% blasts in bone marrow)	18
	RAEB-2 (10–19% blasts in bone marrow)	10
Refractory anaemia with excess blasts in transformation (RAEB-T)	Now part of classification of acute myeloid leukaemia (AML); threshold for AML reduced from 30% blasts in bone marrow to 20%	
Chronic myelomonocytic leukaemia (CMML)	Now considered part of myelodysplastic–myeloproliferative disorder	

Table 8.3 International Prognostic Scoring System for myelodysplastic syndromes

	Score value				
	0	**0.5**	**1**	**1.5**	**2.0**
BM blasts (%)	<5	5–10		11–20	21–30
Karyotype	Good	Intermediate	Poor		
Cytopenias	0 or 1	2 or 3			

BM, bone marrow.
Karyotype:
- Good: normal, −Y, del(5q) or del(20q).
- Intermediate: neither good nor poor abnormalities.
- Poor: complex (≥three abnormalities) or chromosome 7 abnormalities.

Cytopenias: if haemoglobin < 10 g/dL, neutrophils <1.8 × 10⁹/L, platelets < 100 × 10⁹/L.

morphology. It is also important to note that there is a new entity in the WHO classification, namely, MDS associated with isolated 5q−. This is to recognize its excellent median survival, 116 months in one series.

Prognosis

As seen from the above classification, survival can range from months to many years. If a patient has poor risk disease, aggressive management may be offered to them, if appropriate. However, patients with good risk disease will not benefit from aggressive management. Therefore, in 1997, the International Prognostic Scoring System (IPSS) was proposed to risk stratify patients with myelodysplasia. This uses the percentage of bone marrow blasts, the bone marrow karyotype and the number of cytopenias to create an overall score value (Table 8.3). Each score value corresponds to a specific risk group (Table 8.4).

The median survival decreases as the risk group rises from low to high for any given age. For any given risk group, the survival decreases as age increases. Assessment of the IPSS score is therefore important when making management decisions.

Management

In determining the most appropriate management for a given patient, many factors need to be taken into account. These include the patient's age, comorbidities and the severity of their myelodysplasia, as assessed by the IPSS. The availability of a suitable donor for a possible stem cell transplant is also important. Management options include:

1 No active treatment: watch and wait. This may be suitable for patients with mild cytopenias.
2 Supportive care, including transfusion of red cells and platelets, is the mainstay of management of most patients with myelodysplasia. This should take into account patients' symptoms rather than an absolute threshold for transfusion, as well as other comorbid conditions such as chronic cardiorespiratory disease. Iron overload will result from multiple transfusions, and iron chelation therapy should be considered for patients who need regular transfusions but who have a good prognosis, such as those with pure

Table 8.4 Risk stratification and median survival for International Prognostic Scoring System score

Overall score	Risk group	Median survival (years)	Median survival (years)
		(≤60 years old)	(>60 years old)
0	Low	11.8	4.8
0.5–1.0	Intermediate-1	5.2	2.7
1.5–2.0	Intermediate-2	1.8	1.1
≥2.5	High	0.3	0.5

refractory anaemia or isolated 5q− abnormality. This should be considered after the patient has received approximately 25 units of red cells, which is the equivalent of 5 g of iron.

3 It may be possible to reduce transfusion requirements for some patients using erythropoietin injections, with or without granulocyte colony stimulating factor (GCSF). The combination of the two may be particularly effective in refractory anaemia with ringed sideroblasts (RARS).
4 Some 50% of patients with hypoplastic MDS respond to immunosuppression with antilymphocyte globulin (ALG).
5 The investigational drug lenalidomide, a thalidomide analogue, has been shown to reduce or even obviate the need for transfusion in some patients with low risk disease. The effects of lenalidomide were particularly marked in patients with the 5q− syndrome, with 75% of patients achieving complete cytogenetic remission.
6 Hypermethylation of genes involved in cell cycle regulation results in silencing of many genes, especially tumour suppressor genes. DNA methyltransferase inhibitors (hypomethylating agents) can normalize methylating patterns of these genes and may restore differentiation of the abnormal clone. The first drug in this class to be evaluated was azacitidine, shortly followed by decitabine. Azacitidine has been shown to reduce the risk of transformation to leukaemia and improve survival, compared to supportive care alone. Further trials are currently underway.
7 Low-dose cytarabine chemotherapy has been used in high risk MDS with response rates of 15–20%, but this is associated with

considerable toxicity. Although elderly patients tolerate intensive chemotherapy poorly, younger patients with high risk MDS are candidates for AML-type chemotherapy (as per Medical Research Council AML trials). Complete response rates of about 50% can be expected, and patients achieving remission can be considered for a stem cell transplant.

8 Stem cell transplantation remains the only curative treatment for MDS. Patients < 65 years old with high risk disease should be considered for a stem cell transplant. Many factors should be considered, especially the availability of a matched donor and the patient's other comorbid disorders. If a sibling donor is not available, a search for a matched unrelated donor can be initiated. Reduced intensity transplants are less myelosuppressive than standard full intensity transplants, and attempt to harness a 'graft versus leukaemia' effect to eradicate the malignant clone. This results in a reduction in transplant-related mortality and therefore enables patients who otherwise would not be eligible, either on the grounds of age or comorbidity, to receive a transplant.

Further reading

Bennett JM, Catovsky D, Daniel MT *et al.* Proposals for the classification of the myelodysplastic syndromes. *British Journal of Haematology* 1982; **51**: 189–99.

Bowen D, Culligan D, Jowitt S *et al.* Guidelines for the diagnosis and therapy of adult myelodysplastic syndromes *British Journal of Haematology* 2003; **120**: 187–200.

Greenberg P, Cox C, LeBeau MM *et al.* International Scoring System for evaluating prognosis in myelodysplastic syndromes. *Blood* 1997; **89**: 2079–88.

Hellstrom-Lindberg E, Negrin R, Stein R *et al.* Erythroid response to treatment with G-CSF plus erythropoietin for the anaemia of patients with myelodysplastic syndromes: proposal for a predictive model. *British Journal of Haematology* 1997; **99**: 344–51.

Jaffe ES. *Tumours of Haematopoietic and Lymphoid Tissues. World Health Organization Classification of Tumours.* IARC Press, Lyon, 2001.

de Witte T, Suciu S, Verhoef G, *et al.* Intensive chemotherapy followed by allogeneic or autologous stem cell transplantation for patients with myelodysplastic syndromes (MDSs) and acute myeloid leukaemia following MDS. *Blood* 2001; **98**: 2326–31.

CHAPTER 9

Multiple Myeloma and Related Conditions

Charles R J Singer

OVERVIEW

- Consider the diagnosis of myeloma in patients >40 years with symptoms of anaemia, bone pain or recurrent infection or with elevated ESR, hypercalcaemia or renal impairment

- Differentiation of multiple myeloma from monoclonal gammopathy of undetermined significance may be difficult

- No treatment is indicated for monoclonal gammopathy of undetermined significance, but follow-up is essential

- Prognostic factors help identify patients with myeloma in whom treatment may not be necessary (smouldering myeloma), and others in whom aggressive treatment is warranted

- Early chemotherapy may reverse renal impairment and plasmapheresis or dialysis may be appropriate supportive therapy for some patients

- Allogeneic bone marrow transplantation should be considered in myeloma patients <55 years if a compatible sibling donor is available, as this may be curative

- New agents, where available, offer further therapeutic options

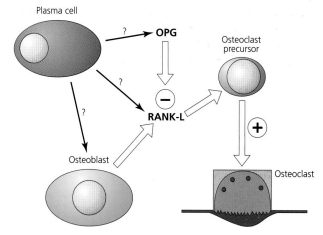

Figure 9.1 Osteoclast activation by myeloma cells. RANK-L, receptor activator of nuclear factor κB ligand (or TRANCE: TNF receptor activation induced cytokine); OPG, osteoprotogerin.

This heterogeneous group of conditions is associated with monoclonal immunoglobulin in serum or urine, and is characterized by disordered proliferation of monoclonal lymphocytes or plasma cells. The clinical phenotypes of these conditions are determined by the rate of accumulation, site and biological properties of both the abnormal cells and the monoclonal protein.

Multiple myeloma

The incidence of myeloma is about 4 per 100 000 in the UK. Myeloma occurs over twice as frequently in African Americans than in white Americans and Europeans, but is much less common among Chinese and Japanese. Myeloma is extremely rare before the age of 40 years but its incidence increases to over 30 per 100 000 in individuals over 80 years. The median age at diagnosis is 69 years, with slight male predominance.

Pathogenesis and clinical features

Myeloma arises in a post-germinal centre B lymphocyte in lymph node or in spleen. Neoplastic cells home into the bone marrow, where the environment facilitates plasma cell proliferation. Interactions between marrow stroma cells and myeloma cells are impor-

tant in disease pathogenesis. Stroma cells produce interleukin (IL)-6, a growth factor for plasma cells, which produce tumour necrosis factor α and IL-1β. These stimulate stroma cell production of the ligand of receptor activator of nuclear factor kappa B (RANK-L). RANK-L promotes osteoclast proliferation and differentiation (Fig. 9.1). Osteoblasts are inhibited in myeloma, as is secretion of osteoprotogerin (OPG; an inhibitor of RANK-L binding and osteoclast formation). As a result, monoclonal plasma cells accumulate in the marrow, causing bone marrow failure and lytic bone destruction (Fig. 9.2).

Most patients have detectable monoclonal paraprotein, usually an intact immunoglobulin (Box 9.1). This is IgG in 60% of patients and IgA in 20–25%. In 15–20% of patients, only immunoglobulin light chains are produced. Free light chains are detectable in urine as Bence–Jones protein. IgD myeloma and non-secretory myeloma are rare. IgE and IgM myelomas are very rare (Fig. 9.3).

The paraprotein may cause hyperviscosity (especially IgA) or protein deposition in renal tubules, resulting in renal failure. Production of normal immunoglobulin is often depressed (immune paresis), which increases susceptibility to infection.

Bone destruction is a characteristic feature, and bone pain is a major cause of morbidity (Box 9.2). This is due to increased bone resorption by osteoclasts and inhibition of osteoblast bone formation causing pronounced bone loss and osteolytic lesions, predisposing

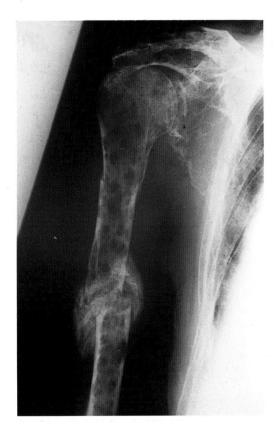

Figure 9.2 Radiograph showing multiple lytic lesions and pathological fractures of the humerus.

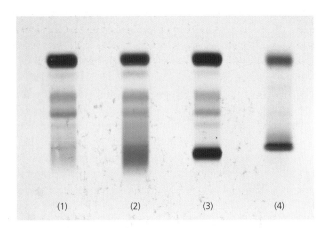

Figure 9.3 Protein electrophoresis strip showing (1) normal plasma, (2) polyclonal hypergammaglobulinaemia, (3) serum paraprotein and (4) Bence–Jones proteinuria and albuminuria.

to pathological fracture. Widespread bone destruction may cause hypercalcaemia and resultant renal failure.

Complex cytogenetic abnormalities are frequently found in myeloma. Fluorescence *in situ* hybridization demonstrates aneuploidy in nearly all cases. These commonly involve chromosome 14q32 (IgH locus) and deletions of chromosome 13, which confer an unfavourable prognosis.

The commonest presentation is bone pain (60%). Symptoms of anaemia, renal failure or infection are frequent. Hyperviscosity (somnolence, impaired vision, purpura and haemorrhage), acute

Box 9.1 Conditions associated with M proteins

Stable production
- Monoclonal gammopathy of undetermined significance
- Smouldering multiple myeloma

Progressive production
- Multiple myeloma (IgG, IgA, free light chains, IgD, IgE, non-secretory, IgM)
- Plasma cell leukaemia
- Solitary plasmacytoma of bone
- Extramedullary plasmacytoma
- Waldenström's macroglobulinaemia (IgM)
- Chronic lymphocytic leukaemia
- Non-Hodgkin's lymphoma
- Primary amyloidosis
- Heavy chain disease

hypercalcaemia, spinal cord compression, neuropathy or amyloidosis may occur. About 20% of patients are asymptomatic and diagnosed by routine blood tests.

Investigations and diagnosis

Myeloma should be suspected in patients aged >40 years with bone pain or fracture, osteoporosis, osteolytic lesions, lethargy, anaemia, red cell rouleaux, raised erythrocyte sedimentation rate (ESR) and plasma viscosity, hypercalcaemia, renal dysfunction, proteinuria, or recurrent infection. It is characterized by the triad of bone marrow plasmacytosis, lytic bone lesions on skeletal radiology, and the presence of M protein in the serum and/or urine (Box 9.3).

Box 9.2 Clinical features of myeloma

Common
- Bone pain and pathological fractures
- Anaemia and bone marrow failure
- Infection due to immune paresis and/or neutropenia
- Renal impairment

Less common
- Acute hypercalcaemia
- Symptomatic hyperviscosity
- Neuropathy
- Amyloidosis
- Coagulopathy

Box 9.3 Diagnostic criteria for multiple myeloma

- Paraprotein in serum and/or urine (NB: no minimum level)
- Bone marrow clonal plasma cells (NB: no minimum level; 5% have <5% plasma cells) or plasmacytoma
- Myeloma-related organ or tissue impairment (end-organ damage):
  - Elevated serum calcium
  - Renal insufficiency
  - Anaemia
  - Bone lesions
  - Others: hyperviscosity, amyloidosis, recurrent bacterial infection

Investigation of a patient with suspected myeloma should include: a full blood count and film, measurement of ESR, plasma viscosity, urea and creatinine concentrations, calcium, phosphate, alkaline phosphatase, uric acid and serum immunoglobulins, serum protein electrophoresis, routine urine analysis, urine electrophoresis for Bence–Jones protein, skeletal survey, and bone marrow aspirate and biopsy (Box 9.4, Fig. 9.4).

Normochromic normocytic anaemia is often present; neutropenia and thrombocytopenia suggest advanced disease (Table 9.1). Rouleaux are usually seen in the blood film, and plasma cells may also be present in about 5% of cases. The ESR and plasma viscosity are usually elevated but are normal in 10% of patients. The serum calcium is increased in up to 20%. Serum alkaline phosphatase is invariably normal, reflecting suppressed osteoblast activity. Raised urea and creatinine occur in 20% and renal impairment, usually due to cast nephropathy, is common. Low serum albumin reflects advanced disease.

Skeletal radiology is a critical investigation and shows lytic lesions, pathological fractures or generalized osteoporosis in 80% of cases.

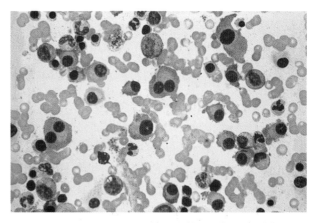

Figure 9.4 Bone marrow aspirate showing infiltrate of abnormal plasma cells (medium power).

Table 9.1 Laboratory findings at diagnosis (proportion of cases)

Normochromic normocytic anaemia	60%
Increased erythrocyte sedimentation rate or plasma viscosity	90%
Serum paraprotein	80%
Urine Bence–Jones protein only	20%
Raised serum calcium concentration	20%
Raised serum creatinine concentration	25%
Proteinuria	70%

Osteoporosis alone is seen in 5–10%. Bone scans are typically negative despite extensive bone damage, and are of no value. Magnetic resonance imaging (MRI) is a sensitive imaging technique for myeloma and is valuable in suspected cord compression (Fig. 9.5).

Box 9.4 **Investigation of patients with suspected myeloma**

Useful screening tests
- Full blood count and film: anaemia often present, film may show rouleaux
- Erythrocyte sedimentation rate or plasma viscosity: raised in the presence of a serum paraprotein
- Urea and creatinine: may identify renal impairment
- Calcium, phosphate, alkaline phosphatase and albumin: may reveal hypercalcaemia or low albumin
- Serum immunoglobulins: to detect immune paresis
- Serum protein electrophoresis: to detect paraprotein
- Routine urinalysis: to detect proteinuria
- Urine electrophoresis for Bence–Jones protein: to detect paraprotein
- X-ray of sites of bone pain: may reveal pathological fracture or lytic lesion(s)

Diagnostic tests
- Bone marrow aspirate: to detect plasma cell infiltration
- Skeletal survey: to identify lytic bone lesions
- Paraprotein typing and quantification: to characterize paraprotein
- Serum free light chains: useful in light chain myeloma and non-secretory myeloma

Tests to establish tumour burden and prognosis
- Serum β-2-microglobulin: measure of tumour load
- Serum C-reactive protein: surrogate measure of interleukin-6
- Serum lactate dehydrogenase: measure of tumour burden
- Serum albumin: low albumin reflects poor prognosis
- Cytogenetics: adds prognostic information

Tests that may be useful in some patients
- Creatinine clearance and 24 hour proteinuria
- Magnetic resonance imaging: not routine but useful in patients with cord compression or solitary plasmacytoma, and is abnormal in 30% of patients with normal skeletal survey
- Computed tomography: where clinically indicated
- Biopsy for amyloid and serum amyloid P scan: where suspected

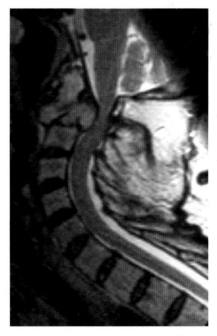

Figure 9.5 Magnetic resonance image showing collapse of second cervical vertebra and narrowing of spinal canal.

Approximately 10% of patients develop primary amyloid, which causes nephrotic syndrome, renal failure, cardiac failure or neuropathy. The extent of amyloid deposition is assessed using serum amyloid P scanning.

The most important differential diagnosis is monoclonal gammopathy of undetermined significance (MGUS), for which no treatment is indicated. No single test differentiates the two conditions reliably. A serum IgG concentration $> 30 \, g/L$ or IgA concentration $> 20 \, g/L$ suggests a diagnosis of myeloma rather than MGUS. The diagnosis of 'smouldering myeloma' is applied to patients in whom paraprotein and bone marrow criteria exist for the diagnosis of myeloma, but no myeloma-related end-organ or tissue impairment occurs and, crucially, the paraprotein remains stable. These patients require close observation but no treatment.

Several prognostic features have been recognized (Box 9.5). Deletion of chromosome 13q is an important adverse feature. Renal impairment is a risk factor, owing to its association with a high tumour burden.

An International Staging System has been devised using serum β-2-microglobulin and albumin concentrations (Table 9.2).

Management and clinical course

Without treatment, patients with multiple myeloma will experience progressive bone damage, anaemia and renal failure. Initial management should prioritize general aspects of care.

Initial treatment should consist of: (i) adequate analgesia – opiates are often necessary, and local radiotherapy to fractures or osteolytic lesions may have dramatic benefit; (ii) rehydration – patients are often dehydrated at presentation, even without hypercalcaemia or renal impairment; (iii) management of hypercalcaemia if present – rehydration, diuresis and bisphosphonate therapy; (iv) management of renal impairment – rehydration and treatment of any hypercalcaemia often have a pronounced effect on abnormal serum chemistry in myeloma, although, in some patients, plasmapheresis and/or dialysis is necessary; (v) treatment of infection – most infections at diagnosis are bacterial and respiratory, and respond to broad spectrum antibiotics; and (vi) chemotherapy (Box 9.6).

Conventional treatment for older patients (> 65 years) is oral melphalan and prednisolone administered at intervals of 4–6 weeks (Box 9.7). This produces $> 50\%$ reduction in paraprotein concentration in 50% of patients. It is well tolerated, but complete response (CR) is rare and maximum response requires 12 months of treatment. Most patients achieve 'plateau phase'; the paraprotein remains

---

Box 9.5 **Adverse prognostic factors at diagnosis**

- Age > 65 years
- Performance status 3 or 4
- Low haemoglobin concentration ($< 8.5 \, g/dL$)
- Hypercalcaemia
- Advanced lytic bone lesions
- High paraprotein production rates (IgG $> 7.0 \, g/dL$; IgA $> 5.0 \, g/dL$; Bence–Jones protein $> 12 \, g/24 \, h$)
- Abnormal renal function
- Low serum albumin concentration ($< 3.0 \, g/dL$)
- High β-2-microglobulin concentration ($> 6 \, mg/mL$)
- High C-reactive protein
- High serum lactate dehydrogenase
- High percentage of bone marrow plasma cells
- Plasmablast morphology
- Adverse cytogenetics: del(13), t(4;14), t(14;16), del(17p), hypoploidy
- Circulating plasma cells in blood film
- High plasma cell proliferative index

Box 9.6 **General aspects of care**

- Pain control
  - Analgesia [caution with non-steroidal anti-inflammatory drugs (NSAIDs)]
  - Local radiotherapy
- Limitation of renal damage
  - Good fluid intake
  - Caution with nephrotoxic drugs including NSAIDs
  - Rapid treatment of hypercalcaemia
- Hypercalcaemia
  - Rehydration
  - Intravenous bisphosphonate
- Bone disease
  - Local radiotherapy
  - Long-term bisphosphonates
  - Fixation of potential fractures
- Cord compression
  - Magnetic resonance imaging scanning to localize lesions
  - Local radiotherapy
- Anaemia
  - Blood transfusion
  - Erythropoietin
- Infection
  - Vigorous antibiotic therapy
  - Annual influenza vaccination
- Hyperviscosity syndrome
  - Plasmapheresis
  - Prompt chemotherapy

Table 9.2 International Staging System

Stage	Findings	Median survival (months)
1	β-2-microglobulin (MG) $< 3.5 \, mg/L$; albumin $\geq 35 \, g/L$	62
2	β-2-MG $< 3.5 \, mg/L$; albumin $< 35 \, g/L$ OR β-2-MG $= 3.5–5.5 \, mg/L$	41
3	β-2-MG $> 5.5 \, mg/L$	29

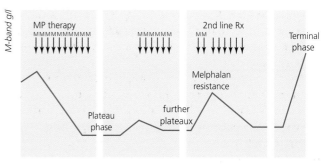

Figure 9.6 Natural history of multiple myeloma after melphalan treatment.

stable without further therapy for a median of 12–18 months. During plateau phase, clinical and laboratory parameters are regularly reviewed to identify progression. If a durable plateau is achieved, further treatment with melphalan may induce another plateau. Median survival is about 3 years. Weekly cyclophosphamide is tolerated by most patients who fail to tolerate melphalan due to cytopenia.

Combination chemotherapeutic regimens produce higher response rates and may improve survival. These may be more effective in younger patients with high tumour loads, but are more toxic in elderly patients. The combination of vincristine, doxorubicin and dexamethasone produces a high response rate (80%), is well tolerated in renal impairment, requires 4–6 months of treatment to achieve maximum response and produces CR in more patients (up to 20%). This treatment is less toxic to haemopoietic progenitors than conventional melphalan or other alkylator-containing regimens and is widely used in patients aged < 65 years in whom autologous stem cell collection is planned.

Patients resistant to first line chemotherapy may respond to thalidomide, the response to which is increased by the addition of dexamethasone and/or cyclophosphamide.

High-dose melphalan and autologous stem cell transplantation after initial treatment with Vincristine, Adriamycin (Doxorobicine) and Dexamethasone (VAD) produces a CR in up to 75% of patients and prolongs survival, but is not curative. It has become standard therapy for patients aged < 65 years. CR is usually associated with prolonged survival. Median duration of CR is 2 years and median overall survival is 5 years.

Allogeneic bone marrow transplantation may cure some patients with myeloma, but carries significant treatment-related morbidity and mortality. It is generally restricted to patients aged < 50 years with a compatible sibling. This treatment offers a 33% chance of durable remission and possible cure, 33% chance of survival with recurrence, and 33% risk of transplant-related mortality.

Plateau phase

Most patients achieve a stable partial response with conventional melphalan therapy, with > 50% reduction in the paraprotein (Fig. 9.6). In plateau phase, cessation of chemotherapy is not followed by a rise in the paraprotein or further signs of progression for many months (median 12–18 months). After high-dose therapy, the plateau phase may be associated with undetectable paraprotein (CR). Maintenance interferon-α may prolong plateau phase by 6 months, but does not improve survival. Maintenance thalidomide may pro-

long response in a significant proportion of patients. Bisphosphonate treatment reduces the rate of further bone damage and may have an additive analgesic effect.

Disease progression

With regular follow-up, serological detection of disease allows therapy to be restarted before new bone damage develops. In many patients, several responses may be re-induced by therapy. Inevitably, myeloma becomes resistant to conventional melphalan. Thalidomide and/or dexamethasone may achieve further disease control. Low-dose cyclophosphamide can be effective palliative treatment in patients unresponsive to or unable to tolerate thalidomide. Local radiotherapy is useful for sites of bone pain (Fig. 9.7). Thalidomide controls myeloma in over 20% of patients with advanced myeloma and, in combination with dexamethasone, in up to 70% of patients previously treated with chemotherapy. The new agents bortezomib

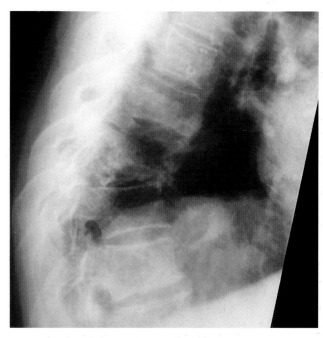

Figure 9.7 Bone pain from mechanical effects of myeloma damage (as in spine shown here) often requires long-term treatment with strong analgesia despite response to chemotherapy.

and Revlimid® can achieve further responses as single agents and in combination with chemotherapy or dexamethasone in patients resistant to other agents. Infection is the most common cause of death.

Conditions related to multiple myeloma

Monoclonal gammopathy of undetermined significance

MGUS is defined by the presence of a paraprotein in a patient without multiple myeloma (Box 9.8), Waldenström's macroglobulinaemia (Box 9.9), amyloidosis, lymphoma, or other related disease (Box 9.10). The prevalence of MGUS is 20 times greater than that of multiple myeloma, and the incidence increases with age (1% over 50 years; 3% over 70 years).

Multiple myeloma, macroglobulinaemia, amyloidosis, or lymphoma ultimately develops in 26% of patients with MGUS, with a cumulative risk of 1–2% per year of follow up (actuarial rate 16% at 10 years).

Solitary plasmacytoma of bone and extramedullary plasmacytoma

About 5% of patients have a single bone or soft tissue (extramedullary) lesion with no evidence of disseminated bone marrow involvement. Generally intact paraprotein is undetectable (up to 70% of cases) or present in low concentration. The serum free light chain

---

Box 9.8 **Diagnostic criteria for MGUS**

- Serum paraprotein <30 g/L
- <10% plasma cells in bone marrow
- No evidence of other B-cell lymphoproliferative disorder
- No myeloma-related organ or tissue impairment (end-organ damage)
- Paraprotein concentration and other results stable on prolonged observation

---

Box 9.9 **Clinical and laboratory features of Waldenström's macroglobulinaemia**

- Fatigue and weight loss
- Anaemia
- Hyperviscosity syndrome (may cause chronic oral or nasal bleeding, visual upset, headache, vertigo, hearing loss, ataxia, somnolence and coma)
- Retinal haemorrhages
- Venous congestion (sausage formation) in retinal veins
- Recurrent infection
- Lymphadenopathy
- Hepatosplenomegaly
- Raised erythrocyte sedimentation rate
- High serum monoclonal IgM concentration
- Lymphoplasmacytoid bone marrow infiltrate

Box 9.10 **Plasma cell leukaemia**

- May be diagnosed when blood plasma cells exceed 2.0×10^9/L
- May occur as a terminal stage in advanced multiple myeloma or as aggressive disease at diagnosis in under 5% of cases
- Bone involvement is often minimal, and the M protein concentration is often low
- Results of treatment are poor; intensive treatment can induce responses and prolong survival

---

assay is abnormal in most patients. Some patients may be cured by radiotherapy (40 cGy). Long-term disease-free survival is achieved in 30% of patients with solitary plasmacytoma of bone and in 60% with extramedullary plasmacytoma. Both should be monitored long-term. Further plasmacytoma or myeloma may develop. MRI may identify bone lesions undetectable by X-ray. Median survival is over 10 years.

Waldenström's macroglobulinaemia

Waldenström's macroglobulinaemia is caused by proliferation of lymphoid cells that produce monoclonal IgM. The median age at presentation is 63 years, and over 60% are men. Many clinical features are due to hyperviscosity. Weakness, fatigue and bleeding are common, followed by visual upset, weight loss, recurrent infection, dyspnoea, heart failure and neurological symptoms. Bone pain is rare.

The ESR is greatly elevated. If the plasma viscosity exceeds 4 centipoise (cP), symptoms of hyperviscosity are frequent. All patients have an IgM paraprotein. Monoclonal light chains may be present in the urine. Trephine biopsy often shows extensive infiltration with plasmacytoid lymphocytes.

Symptomatic hyperviscosity requires urgent plasmapheresis. Chlorambucil for 7–14 days every 4 weeks usually reduces bone marrow lymphocytosis, serum IgM concentration and plasma viscosity, and improves symptoms. Median survival is about 5 years. Fludarabine is an effective alternative and is good second line therapy. Rituximab induces responses in up to 75%.

Other related conditions

Chronic lymphocytic leukaemia and low grade non-Hodgkin's lymphomas may produce small amounts of monoclonal IgG or IgM. This has no prognostic importance. Primary amyloidosis is associated with a low level paraprotein in 85% of cases and abnormal serum free light chains. The 'heavy chain diseases' are rare lymphoproliferative disorders in which abnormal cells excrete only parts of immunoglobulin heavy chains (γ, α, or μ).

Further reading

Dispenzieri A, Kyle RA. Multiple myeloma: clinical features and indications for therapy. *Best Practice and Research. Clinical Haematology* 2005; **18**: 553–68.

Greipp P, San Miguel JF, Durie BG *et al*. International staging system for multiple myeloma. *Journal of Clinical Oncology* 2005; **20**: 3412–20.

Harousseau J-L, Moreau P, Attal M *et al*. Stem cell transplantation in multiple myeloma. *Best Practice and Research. Clinical Haematology* 2005; **18**: 603–18.

International Myeloma Working Group. Criteria for the classification of the monoclonal gammopathies, multiple myeloma and related disorders. *British Journal of Haematology* 2003; **121**: 749–57.

Johnson S, Oscier D, Leblond V. Waldenstrom's macroglobulinaemia. *Blood Reviews* 2002; **16**: 175.

Kyle RA, Rajkumar SV. Multiple myeloma. *New England Journal of Medicine* 2004; **351**: 1060–77.

UK Myeloma Forum, Nordic Myeloma Study Group and British Committee for Standards in Haematology. Guidelines on the diagnosis and management of multiple myeloma 2005. *British Journal of Haematology* 2006; **132**: 410–51.

UK Myeloma Forum. Guidelines on the diagnosis and management of solitary plasmacytoma of bone and solitary extramedullary plasmacytoma. *British Journal of Haematology* 2004; **124**: 717–26

CHAPTER 10

Bleeding Disorders, Thrombosis and Anticoagulation

David M Keeling

OVERVIEW

Blood within the circulation must remain fluid, but if a blood vessel is damaged, localized coagulation must take place to prevent loss of blood. When there is injury to a blood vessel, a series of events is initiated which results in controlled haemostasis. This involves:

1 Local vasoconstriction

2 Adhesion and aggregation of platelets

3 Activation of the clotting cascade to form a fibrin clot

4 Activation of coagulation inhibitors to ensure coagulation is restricted to the site of injury

5 Late fibrinolysis to restore patency of the vessel.

These complex interacting systems can be disturbed by inherited or acquired factors, resulting in bleeding or thrombotic disorders

Bleeding disorders

The approach to a patient with a suspected bleeding disorder involves medical history, examination, coagulation screening tests and specialist coagulation tests.

History and examination

When assessing a patient for a possible bleeding disorder, a good history is of paramount importance (Box 10.1). Is the bleeding mucocutaneous (Box 10.2) [often seen in platelet defects and von Willebrand disease(VWD)], or into joints and muscles (often seen

---

Box 10.1 History in a suspected bleeding disorder

- Type of bleeding: mucocutaneous, haemarthroses/muscle hae-matomas
- Severity of bleeding: blood transfusions, anaemia
- Previous tests of the haemostatic system
  - Operations
  - Dental extractions
  - Trauma
  - Childbirth
- Age of onset
- Family history
- Other medical problems
- Drugs: aspirin, non-steroidal anti-inflammatory drugs

Box 10.2 History suggestive of mucocutaneous bleeding

- Prolonged epistaxis
- Cutaneous haemorrhage and bruising with minimal or no apparent trauma
- Prolonged bleeding from trivial wounds
- Oral cavity bleeding
- Spontaneous gastrointestinal bleeding
- Menorrhagia not associated with structural lesions of the uterus

---

in coagulation factor deficiencies)? The severity must be assessed; did it result in anaemia or a blood transfusion? These objective findings are important, as many normal people report that they 'bruise easily'. Particular attention must be paid to previous tests of the haemostatic system, for example, operations, dental extractions, trauma and childbirth. The age of onset and a family history are important to address the issue of whether the condition is likely to be inherited or acquired. Menorrhagia beginning from the menarche is much more likely to be due to an inherited coagulation defect than is menorrhagia starting later in life. If there is a family history, the mode of inheritance is important, for example, X-linked recessive inheritance suggests haemophilia A or B. Any other medical problems must be identified along with the use of any drugs which may affect haemostasis, such as aspirin or non-steroidal anti-inflammatory drugs. The common acquired causes of a coagulopathy, vitamin K deficiency, disseminated intravascular coagulation (DIC) and liver disease, must be considered, as well as conditions that may be mistaken for a coagulopathy (Box 10.3). The examination looks for evidence of bleeding and bruising but is mainly directed at detecting systemic disease.

Box 10.3 Conditions which may be mistaken for a coagulopathy

- Henoch–Schonlein vasculitis
- Vitamin C deficiency
- Steroid purpura/Cushing's disease
- Amyloid in the skin vessels
- Ehlers–Danlos/pseudoxanthoma elasticum
- Cryoglobulinaemia

Laboratory investigation

Most important bleeding disorders can be excluded if the full blood count (FBC), prothrombin time (PT), activated partial thromboplastin time (APTT), thrombin time (TT) or fibrinogen, and closure time on the PFA100 platelet function analyser or bleeding time are normal. However, it is important to realize that mild VWD and some mild platelet defects, such as storage pool disease, can be missed by these screening tests. If a bleeding disorder is strongly suspected, factor VIII, von Willebrand factor (VWF) activity and VWF antigen should be measured, and platelet aggregation and platelet nucleotide measurements performed. If all these tests are normal in a case with a convincing history, deficiencies of factor XIII and α2-antiplasmin should be considered (Box 10.4).

Figure 10.1 shows a simplified version of the coagulation cascade. This representation, although non-physiological, enables us to interpret the coagulation screening tests (Table 10.1). Heparin can some-

Box 10.4 Investigations in suspected abnormal bleeding

Screening tests
- Full blood count
- Prothrombin time
- Activated partial thromboplastin time
- Thrombin time or fibrinogen
- PFA100 closure or bleeding time

Other first line investigations
- Factor VIII, von Willebrand factor (VWF) activity, VWF antigen
- Platelet aggregation
- Platelet nucleotides

Second line investigations
- Factor XIII
- α2-antiplasmin

Table 10.1 Interpretation of coagulation screening tests

Result	Cause
PT prolonged, APTT normal	Deficiency of factor VII (seen in early vitamin K deficiency/oral anticoagulation or liver disease)
PT normal, APTT prolonged	Deficiency of factors VIII, IX, XI (or the contact factors) Lupus anticoagulant
PT prolonged, APTT prolonged TT normal	Deficiencies of factors II, V, X Vitamin K deficiency/oral anticoagulation Liver disease
TT prolonged	Afibrinogenaemia* Heparin* DIC

*See text. APTT, activated partial thromboplastin time; DIC, disseminated intravascular coagulation; PT, prothrombin time; TT, thrombin time.

times prolong APTT (and TT) without prolonging PT, and occasionally a low fibrinogen may not be detected by PT and APTT (hence the importance of either TT or a direct measurement of fibrinogen).

Congenital bleeding disorders

Haemophilia A (factor VIII deficiency, with a frequency of 1 in 5000 male births) and haemophilia B (factor IX deficiency, 1 in 25 000 male births) are phenotypcally identical X-linked recessive disorders. Patients with severe haemophilia (< 1% factor VIII or IX) have spontaneous bleeding into muscles and joints that can lead to a crippling arthropathy (Fig. 10.2). Patients with moderate (1–5%) and mild (> 5%) factor levels usually bleed only after trauma or surgery. Management is usually undertaken in specialist haemophilia centres. Mild haemophilia A will respond to desmopressin, otherwise clotting factors are given. In developed countries, these are increasingly being replaced by recombinant coagulation factors to avoid plasma-derived infections.

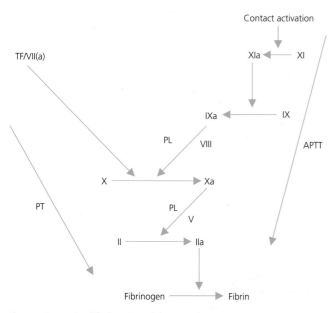

Figure 10.1 A simplified version of the coagulation cascade. TF, tissue factor; PT, prothrombin time; PL, phospholipid; APTT, activated partial thromboplastin time.

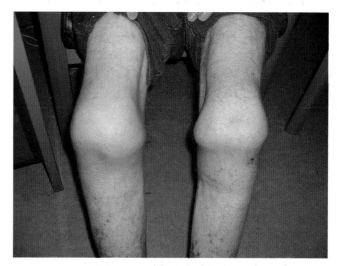

Figure 10.2 Knee arthropathy in haemophilia.

VWD is a common disorder caused by a reduction or structural abnormality of VWF. VWF has the dual role of promoting platelet adhesion to exposed collagen and protecting factor VIII in the circulation. In VWD, the main defect is the resulting abnormal platelet function and is manifest by mucocutaneous bleeding. Menorrhagia is common in affected women. Most cases are mild, with significant bleeding only occurring after a haemostatic challenge. Inheritance is usually autosomal dominant. Most patients with mild disease respond to desmopressin, but clotting factor concentrates are sometimes needed.

Acquired bleeding disorders

The common acquired coagulopathies are DIC, liver disease and vitamin K deficiency (Box 10.5). DIC occurs when a pathological stimulus to coagulation results in widespread microvascular thrombosis. This in turn results in a consumption of coagulation factors and platelets and a stimulation of fibrinolysis, which results in concurrent bleeding. It can be induced by conditions such as sepsis, trauma, malignancy, obstetric complications and severe transfusion reactions. In liver disease, there may be loss of synthetic function, and, as the proteins of the coagulation cascade are synthesized in the liver, this results in a coagulopathy often exacerbated by thrombocytopenia. An inadequate dietary intake or malabsorption of vitamin K will give a coagulopathy due to failure of γ-carboxylate factors II, VII, IX and X.

Venous thromboembolism

Venous thromboembolism – deep vein thrombosis (DVT) and pulmonary embolism – is due to a combination of blood stasis and hypercoagulability. The predisposing factors are shown in Box 10.6. In addition, a previous history of venous thromboembolism is a strong

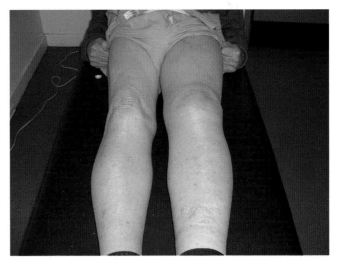

Figure 10.3 Deep vein thrombosis.

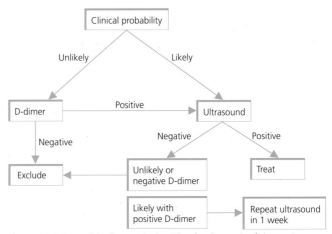

Figure 10.4 A possible diagnostic algorithm for diagnosis of deep vein thrombosis.

Box 10.5 **Common acquired coagulopathies**

- Disseminated intravascular coagulation
- Liver disease
- Vitamin K deficiency

Box 10.6 **Risk factors for venous thromboembolism**

- Age
- Immobilization and paresis
- Surgery and trauma
- Malignancy
- Pregnancy and the puerperium
- The combined oral contraceptive pill
- Hormone replacement therapy
- The inherited thrombophilias
- Antiphospholipid antibodies
- Raised coagulation factors, e.g. factor VIII
- Family history of venous thromboembolism
- Serious illness

risk factor as this is a recurrent condition. Obesity, varicose veins and smoking are only weak risk factors.

Diagnosis is often made using a diagnostic algorithm which involves clinical examination (Fig. 10.3), D-dimer (fibrin degradation fragment) testing and imaging investigations such as ultrasound. A typical diagnostic algorithm for DVT is shown in Fig. 10.4.

The inherited thrombophilias

The natural anticoagulant pathways are shown in Fig. 10.5. Many of the coagulation proteins are serine proteases. Antithrombin is a member of a family of proteins known as serine protease inhibitors or serpins. It forms a one-to-one stoichiometric complex with serine proteases, thus neutralizing them. As its name implies, its main effect is to neutralize thrombin, although it does also have significant inhibitory activity against factor Xa.

Activated protein C acts as a natural anticoagulant by cleaving the two cofactors in the coagulation pathway, factors V and VIII. To do this it needs its own cofactor, protein S. Proteins C and S are

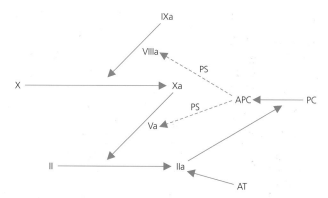

Figure 10.5 The natural anticoagulants. APC, activated protein C; AT, antithrombin; PC, protein C; PS, protein S.

both vitamin K-dependent proteins. The zymogen (inactive precursor form) protein C is activated by thrombin in the presence of an endothelial cell cofactor, thrombomodulin. It has been known for some time that deficiencies of antithrombin, protein C or protein S predispose to thrombosis. Heterozygotes for these deficiencies with 50% of normal levels are at risk, and therefore the thrombotic tendency is inherited in an autosomal dominant fashion.

Until 1993, these three deficiencies were the only well characterized forms of inherited thrombophilia (Table 10.2). In 1993, the phenomenon of resistance to activated protein C was described. One year later, the molecular defect was identified as a G→A substitution at nucleotide position 1691 in factor V (FV). This results in the arginine at position 506 being replaced by a glutamine. Using the single letter amino acid code, the mutant FV can therefore be written as FV R506Q, but is more often referred to as FV Leiden (Fig. 10.6). Normally, FV is inactivated by an initial cleavage of the peptide bond at arginine 506, but the mutant FV is resistant to activated protein C. FV Leiden is present in 5% of the population, but is found in 20% of all cases of DVT, as it increases the risk of DVT approximately 4–7-fold.

Table 10.2 The heritable thrombophilias

Condition	Prevalence
Antithrombin deficiency	1 in 3000
Protein C deficiency	1 in 300
Protein S deficiency	1 in 300
Factor V Leiden	1 in 20
Prothrombin G20210A	1 in 80

Factor V Leiden (R506Q)

505	506	507
Arg	**Arg**	Gly
AGG	C**G**A	GGA
	↓	
AGG	C**A**A	GGA
Arg	**Gln**	Gly

Figure 10.6 The G→A point mutation results in the arginine at the protein C cleavage site being replaced by glutamine.

Shortly afterwards, it was discovered that a mutation in the 3′ untranslated region of the prothrombin gene, which is present in 1–2% of the population, is associated with an approximately three-fold increased risk of venous thromboembolism. The mechanism seems to be higher prothrombin levels in individuals with the mutation.

It is not recommended that all cases of venous thromboembolism are investigated for inherited thrombophilia, however (Box 10.6); the criteria for those whom we should investigate are shown in Box 10.7.

In addition to testing for inherited thrombophilia, consideration should also be given to testing for antiphospholipid antibodies, which are acquired and are associated with both venous and arterial disease. It is important to recognize that the inherited forms of thrombophilia are associated with venous thrombosis but not arterial disease.

Treatment of venous thromboembolism

Heparin

The initial treatment is anticoagulation with heparin. Heparin is a mixture of glycosaminoglycan chains of varying length. Low molecular weight heparin (LMWH), which has a mixture of shorter chains, is now the usual treatment. A specific pentasaccharide chain in the heparin chain binds to antithrombin and dramatically improves its ability to inhibit thrombin and factor Xa. The dose of LMWH can be calculated by body weight and given subcutaneously once a day without any monitoring or dose adjustment.

Warfarin

After the diagnosis has been made, oral anticoagulation with warfarin can be commenced. Warfarin is a vitamin K antagonist, which prevents necessary post-translational modification of factors II, VII, IX and X. Warfarin therapy is monitored by the international normalized ratio (INR; a manipulation of the prothrombin time to take account of the reagent used). For the treatment of venous thromboembolism, the target INR is usually 2.5 (range 2.0–3.0). Warfarin is continued for 5 days, or until the INR is > 2.0 on two consecutive days, whichever is the longer.

Further reading

Investigation and management of heritable thrombophilia. *British Journal of Haematology* 2001; **114**: 512–28.

Guidelines on oral anticoagulation: third edition. *British Journal of Haematology* 1998; **101**: 374–87.

Buller HR, Agnelli G, Hull RD, Hyers TM, Prins MH, Raskob GE. Antithrombotic therapy for venous thromboembolic disease: the Seventh ACCP Conference on Antithrombotic and Thrombolytic Therapy. *Chest* 2004; **126** (Suppl): 401S-28S.

Keeling DM, Mackie IJ, Moody A, Watson HG. The diagnosis of deep vein thrombosis in symptomatic outpatients and the potential for clinical assessment and D-dimer assays to reduce the need for diagnostic imaging. *British Journal of Haematology* 2004; **124**: 15–25.

Mannucci PM. Treatment of von Willebrand's disease. *New England Journal of Medicine* 2004; **351**: 683–94.

Mannucci PM, Tuddenham EG. The hemophilias – from royal genes to gene therapy. *New England Journal of Medicine* 2001; **344**: 1773–9.

CHAPTER 11

Lymphoproliferative Disorders Including Chronic Lymphocytic Leukaemia

Bronwen Shaw, Simon O'Connor, Andrew P Haynes

OVERVIEW

- Lymphomas are a clinically heterogeneous group of haematological malignancies

- Accurate histopathological diagnosis is important and often requires specialised techniques. Access to a dedicated haematopathology service and specialist haematopathologist is essential

- Chemotherapy, radiotherapy, transplantation and biological therapies may all be relevant. A large portfolio of NCRI studies is available. It is critical that individual cases are discussed by relevant experts in the context of a structured MDT

- Scientific understanding of these malignancies is rapidly advancing and gene profiling highlighting further heterogeneity amongst standard histological types which are often of prognostic value and may soon be relevant for treatment selection

- The development of biological therapy is well advanced in some lymphomas. A good example is the monoclonal antibody Rituximab which has activity against a wide range of B cell tumours and benefits for survival such that its routine use in appropriate situations has been approved by NICE

To the uninitiated, the lymphoproliferative disorders are a confusing group of human tumours. They usually involve the lymph nodes but may also present in extranodal lymphatic tissue in the spleen, marrow, lung or gastrointestinal tract. Some aspects of their biology can mimic that of normal lymphocytes with circulating 'leukaemic phase' disease and infiltration of other tissues, for example, liver, skin, brain, salivary glands and thyroid. In general, 85% of lymphoproliferative disorders are B cell in origin, in contrast to the situation in normal blood, where over 90% of lymphocytes are T cells. Histologically, lymphoproliferative disorders are divided into Hodgkin's lymphoma (HL), characterized by the presence of Reed–Sternberg cells, and non-Hodgkin's lymphoma (NHL). The NHLs are further classified by their growth rate. Low grade NHL grows slowly, and hence may have been present for many years, can be widely disseminated with minimal symptoms, does not always need but can usually be easily controlled by treatment, and is associated with long-term survival. High grade disease, such as diffuse large cell lymphoma, grows rapidly and is fatal if untreated, but shows a high response and cure rate. In between these two is a small group of intermediate grade diseases, which grow more rapidly than low but not as fast as high grade disease; the best example is mantle cell lymphoma (MCL). Although, historically, chronic lymphocytic leukaemia (CLL) has been considered as a separate entity, it is in fact biologically a low grade NHL that displays leukaemic phase overspill from marrow involvement.

Incidence

Non-Hodgkin's lymphoma

NHL has an incidence of 16 per 100 000 per annum, representing 4% of all cancers. It is more common in males than females, in urban than rural communities, and in white than black patients. The median age is 65–70 years. The incidence of NHL has been increasing in Western countries by >3% per year since the 1970s. The reasons for this are largely unexplained.

Chronic lymphocytic leukaemia

CLL is the most common type of leukaemia in the Western world (4 per 100 000). The median age of presentation is 65 years.

Hodgkin's lymphoma

HL has an incidence of 2–3 per 100 000 per annum. It has a bimodal age distribution; in the 15–34-year age group it is the second most common tumour in males and the fourth in females, and a later smaller peak occurs around the age of 65 years.

Epidemiology and aetiology

There is a marked difference in the geographical distribution of different subtypes of lymphoproliferative disorders; for example, in the Western world, follicular lymphoma is common whereas natural killer cell/T cell (NK/T) tumours are less so; the opposite situation is found in Japan and the Far East. In contrast, CLL is very common in the West, but is much rarer in China and the Far East.

There are a number of well defined aetiological factors in the development of lymphomas.

Immunodeficiency

In human immunodeficiency virus (HIV) infection, a 60-fold increased risk of lymphoproliferative disorders is expressed by the occurrence of aggressive B-cell lymphomas, including Burkitt's lymphoma and HL. Similarly, in patients receiving long-term immune suppression following solid organ transplantation, a significant increased risk of aggressive B-cell tumours is seen (post-transplant lymphoproliferative disease; PTLD). Patients with congenital immunodeficiency state, for example, Ataxia Telangiectasia, are also at higher risk of developing lymphoproliferative disorders.

Chronic immune stimulation

- Human T-cell lymphotrophic virus is associated with adult T-cell leukaemia/lymphoma in a small proportion of cases infected with the virus.
- Epstein–Barr virus is associated with Burkitt's lymphoma and PTLD.
- *Helicobacter pylori* has been found in mucosa-associated lymphoid tissue (MALT) lymphomas in the stomach and gut.
- Rheumatoid arthritis is associated with a 40-fold increased risk of Bcell NHL.
- Chronic sialadenitis in Sjögren's disease and thyroiditis in Hashimoto's disease are associated with marginal zone B cell NHLs.

Familial aggregation

This may be due to genetic predisposition within the immune system, shared environmental exposure, or both. Other aetiological agents have been much less conclusively linked to lymphoproliferative disorders; however, chronic exposure to pesticides, fertilizers, certain foods and hair-colouring agents has been associated with increased risk.

Classification

The basis of classification systems is to take into account a number of properties of the tumour. These include: morphology, immunophenotype, genotype, normal cell counterpart and clinical features (site of origin, aggressiveness and prognosis).

Morphology is the mainstay of diagnosis. Immunophenotyping in circulating cells, marrow or tissue sections can be very useful in distinguishing reactive from malignant states and subclassifying the lymphoma type. Genetic studies of DNA/RNA or chromosomes may be helpful in establishing an accurate diagnosis and subclassifying disease, and can give prognostic information. These elements are combined in the World Health Organization classification (Table 11.1), which is the internationally applied standard in diagnostic haematopathology laboratories (Figs 11.1–11.3).

Presenting features

The lymphoproliferative diseases may present in a number of different ways.

- Incidental finding: for example, a raised lymphocyte count (such as in CLL) in an otherwise well patient.
- Lymphadenopathy: this may be localized or generalized. The nodes are characteristically painless, rubbery and non-tender. Unlike solid tumours, even relatively large lymph node masses are usually asymptomatic. Compression of the ureters may cause

Table 11.1 World Health Organization classification (major categories) of lymphoma

Classification	Frequency (%)	5-year survival (%)
B lineage		
• Diffuse large B-cell lymphoma	30.6	40 (15 to >90)
• Follicular lymphoma	22.0	60 (20 to >90)
• Marginal zone B-cell lymphoma/mucosa-associated lymphoid tissue	7.6	70 (60 to >90)
• Chronic lymphocytic leukaemia/small lymphocytic lymphoma	6.7	>50 (20 to >90)
• Mantle cell lymphoma	6.0	25
• Primary mediastinal large B-cell lymphoma	2.4	70
• Burkitt's/Burkitt-like lymphoma	2.5	85
T lineage		
• Peripheral T-cell lymphoma	7.0	25
• Anaplastic large cell lymphoma	2.4	70 (15 to >90)
• Lymphoblastic lymphoma	1.7	30
Hodgkin's lymphoma (HL) (30% of lymphomas)		
• Nodular lymphocyte-predominant HL	5	>90
• Classical HL	95	>80
• Nodular sclerosis classical HL		
• Lymphocyte-rich classical HL		
• Mixed cellularity classical HL		
• Lymphocyte-depleted classical HL		

Colour key:

High grade
Intermediate grade
Low grade

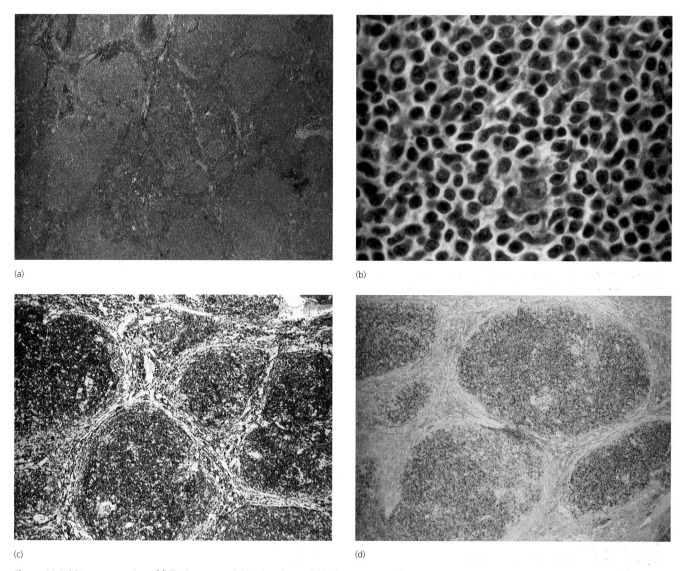

(a)

(b)

(c)

(d)

Figure 11.1 (a) Low power view of follicular non-Hodgkin's lymphoma; (b) high power view of centrocytes within follicles; (c) neoplastic centrocytes stained for Bcl-2 expression; (d) neoplastic centrocytes stained for CD10 to confirm germinal centre origin.

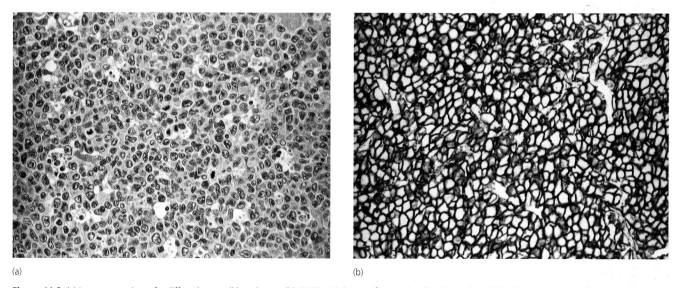

(a)

(b)

Figure 11.2 (a) Low power view of a diffuse large cell lymphoma; (b) CD20 staining confirming B-cell origin and suitability for therapy, including the anti-CD20 monoclonal antibody rituximab.

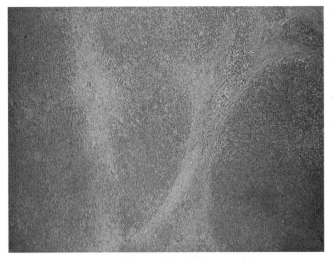

(a)

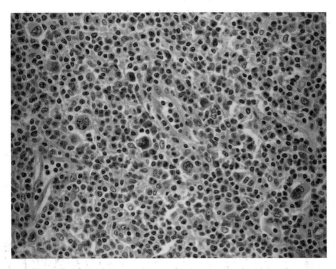

(b)

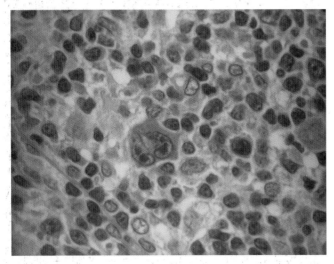

(c)

Figure 11.3 (a) Low power view showing bands of fibrosis in Hodgkin's lymphoma; (b) low power view showing large mononuclear Reed–Sternberg cells in a background of reactive cells with prominent eosinophils; (c) high power view of a classical binucleate Reed–Sternberg cell.

hydronephrosis, or of the venous return from a limb may cause oedema.
- Hepatosplenomegaly.
- Mediastinal involvement: this may present as chest symptoms or superior vena cava syndrome (see page 65).
- Constitutional symptoms ('B' symptoms): fevers, night sweats, loss of weight (>10% of body weight in 6 months). HL may also present with pruritis or, rarely, alcohol-induced pain in lymph node masses.
- Bone marrow failure: symptoms due to anaemia, thrombocytopenia or leucopenia.
- Any other organ may be involved and a high index of suspicion is often needed in these cases (for example, nasopharyngeal involvement in NK lymphomas, gastrointestinal involvement by MALT lymphomas, skin in T-cell lymphomas).

Investigations

In those presenting with a suspected lymphoproliferative disorder, investigations should include those important in making the diagnosis, those important in staging the disease (Table 11.2), assessing prognosis (Table 11.3), and those assessing the overall condition of the patient (for example, to assess the appropriateness of a certain treatment strategy).
- Histology is critical to the diagnosis of lymphoproliferative disorders. This can be obtained from a biopsy of affected lymph nodes or extranodal site (for example, bone marrow, liver, skin, etc). Wherever possible, a node biopsy should be performed to give an adequate volume of material to assess architectural context. Fine needle aspirates are usually inadequate to make an accurate diagnosis. Tests will include immunohistochemistry to look for particular markers on the cell, which will aid classification.
- Full blood count: this may show a lymphocytosis (for example, CLL, mantle cell lymphoma), pancytopenia (bone marrow failure), lymphopenia (HL, HIV-related lymphoma), eosinophilia (HL or T-cell lymphoma) or neutrophilia (HL). Immunophenotyping can be performed.
- Bone marrow investigation: this can include morphological examination, immunophenotyping and assessment of genetic factors by chromosome analysis or fluorescence *in situ* hybridization (FISH).

Table 11.2 Staging of lymphomas (Ann Arbor)

Stage	Criteria
I	Single lymph node region or single extralymphatic site
II	Two or more lymph node regions on the same side of the diaphragm; localized contiguous involvement of only one extralymphatic site and lymph node region (stage IIE)
III	Involvement of lymph node regions on both sides of the diaphragm; may include the spleen
IV	Disseminated involvement of one or more extralymphatic organs with or without lymph node involvement

A, no systemic symptoms; B, unexplained fever of at least 38°C, night sweats, weight loss (>10% body weight in 6 months). Any stage may be A or B depending on the absence or presence of constitutional symptoms.

Table 11.3 Poor prognostic factors at diagnosis

Parameter	Aggressive lymphoma (IPI)	Follicular lymphoma (FLIPI)	CLL	Advanced HL (Hasenclever Index/ IPS)*
Age	>60 years	>60 years		>45 years
Lactate dehydrogenase	Raised	Raised	Raised†	
Stage	III/IV	III/IV	Binet B/C Rai II–IV	IV
WHO performance status	>2	>4		
Extranodal sites	>1		Diffuse pattern of BM involvement	
Gender			Male	Male
Albumin				<40 g/L
Haematological		Hb < 12 g/dL	Abnormal lymphocyte morphology	Hb < 10.5 g/dL; WCC >15×10⁹/L; lymphocytes <0.6×10⁹/L
Other		≥4 nodal sites of disease	High CD38 expression; unmutated IgVH gene ZAP-70 expression	

* Presence of each adverse factor reduces the probability of disease-free survival by 8%.
† As well as other serum markers, for example, β-2-microglobulin. CLL, chronic lymphocytic leukaemia; FL, follicular lymphoma; Hb, haemoglobin; HL, Hodgkin's lymphoma; IPI, International Prognostic Index; IPS, International Prognostic Score; WCC, white cell count; WHO, World Health Organization.

- Immunophenotyping: this can be performed on peripheral blood or bone marrow samples (or other fluid such as cerebrospinal or pleural fluid) and can be extremely useful in the diagnosis of certain lymphoproliferative disorders. In particular, immunophenotyping is helpful in the differential diagnosis of the low grade lymphoproliferative disorders and CLL.

- Cytogenetics: recognized recurrent chromosomal abnormalities can be helpful in establishing/confirming the diagnosis of a particular subtype of lymphoproliferative disorder (Table 11.2). This investigation is usually performed on the bone marrow sample and may be carried out by a number of techniques including polymerase chain reaction and FISH.

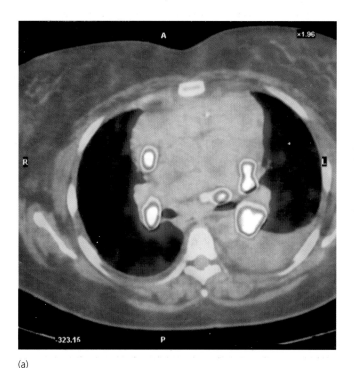

(a)

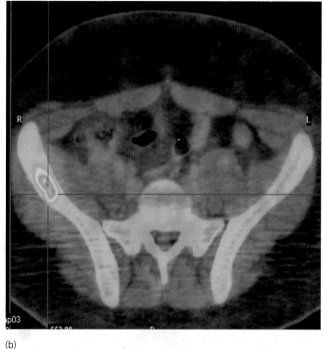

(b)

Figure 11.4 (a) Computed tomography (CT)/positron emission tomography (PET) scan after treatment showing multiple mediastinal nodes, some of which are PET positive indicating residual active disease; (b) CT/PET scan at diagnosis indicating a focus of disease activity in the right iliac wing.

- Serum markers: for example, erythrocyte sedimentation rate, β-2-microglobulin.
- HIV and other viral tests: as mentioned above, viruses may be implicated in the pathogenesis of many of the lymphomas. In addition, certain lymphomas are more common in patients with HIV [for example, Burkitt's lymphoma, primary central nervous system (CNS) lymphoma].
- Chemistry: renal function, liver function, uric acid, calcium.
- Immunoglobulins: a paraprotein may be present (for example, CLL, marginal zone or lymphoplasmacytic NHL) and there may be co-existing immunoparesis.
- Imaging: chest X-ray, computed tomography, magnetic resonance imaging, positron emission tomography (PET) scan (Fig. 11.4). PET, with fluoro-deoxyglucose, is increasingly being used in patients with lymphoma. Its applications include staging, response assessment and prediction of relapse. Currently, its widespread use is hampered by cost and the absence of data from large, well run randomized clinical trials

Access to specialist haematopathology laboratories to confirm the diagnosis should be available.

Further/future investigations

Although not yet in routine clinical use, gene microarrays are being extensively studied in the lymphoproliferative disorders. They have been shown to be helpful in many areas including diagnosis, staging and prognosis and, in addition, in the understanding of the molecular processes that underlie the pathology in specific diseases.

Prognosis

The prognosis in individual patients is based on a number of factors, which differ depending on the disease subtype (Table 11.3). In general, these systems are based on simple, readily measurable clinical parameters, which are surrogates for biology and, as such, predict general rather than individual behaviour. Gene expression profiling (GEP) has begun to add additional biological information

(Table 11.4, Fig. 11.5) but is not yet in routine diagnostic practice. In aggressive B-cell NHL, two types of disease can be distinguished by GEP; one originating from germinal centre B cells (GCB) with a 5-year survival rate of > 70%, and a non-GCB group with a 5-year survival rate of < 15%.

Treatment

A diagnosis of cancer is usually a great shock to the patient, even if he or she has suspected it. The way in which the diagnosis is relayed will have a large impact on the patient's understanding and cooperation with treatment. In addition, the ability of the patient to trust the clinician will be formed at this stage.

Patients should be offered access to resources such as pamphlets, support groups and (reputable) websites. Specialist nurses with specific knowledge of lymphoma are a valuable resource. Some patients may benefit from meeting other patients with the same diagnosis.

In general, patients should be assessed and managed by clinicians familiar with lymphoproliferative disorders and chemo/radiotherapy. Inclusion in a clinical trial may be appropriate; the National Cancer Research Institute Lymphoma Trials group offers a wide portfolio. Discussion of treatment strategies in a multidisciplinary meeting is crucial.

Prior to deciding on the type of treatment, it is important for both the clinician and patient to understand and agree on what is the intended outcome of therapy. This will depend on many factors, including the patient's age, performance status and comorbidity, as well as the kinetics of the underlying disease (indolent or aggressive). Approaches may aim to cure or control the disease, to control symptoms or to palliate.

In general, the high grade malignancies tend to act aggressively, require high-dose, high-intensity therapy and may be curable. It is important for patients to understand that complete remission does not guarantee cure; disease that is below the level of detection may still be present at the end of treatment and cause relapse.

Table 11.4 Recognized chromosomal translocations found in non-Hodgkin's lymphoma (including frequency and most reliable method of detection)

Type of lymphoma	Mutation	Gene involved	Percentage with translocation	Optimum testing method
DLBCL	t(3;4)	*BCL-6*/other	> 30 (BCL-6)	
	t(14;18)	IgH/*BCL-2*	15–20	FISH, PCR
Follicular	t(14;18)	IgH/*BCL-2*	~85	PCR, FISH
MZL	t(11;18)	*AP12/MALT1*	Up to 40	FISH, PCR
	t(1;14)	*BCL10*/IgH	Rare	FISH, PCR
	t(14;18)	IgH/*MALT1*	15–20	FISH
MCL	t(11;14)	*BCL-1*/IgH	100	FISH, PCR
Burkitt's lymphoma	t(8;14)	*c-myc*/IgH	80	FISH
	t(8;2)	*c-myc*/Igκ	20	FISH
	t(8;22)	*c-myc*/Igλ		FISH
T-cell anaplastic	t(2;5)	*ALK/NPM*	~50	FISH, RT-PCR

CLL, chronic lymphocytic leukaemia/small lymphocytic lymphoma; DLBCL, diffuse large B-cell lymphoma; FISH, fluorescence *in situ* hybridization; MCL, mantle cell lymphoma; MZL, marginal zone lymphoma; PCR, polymerase chain reaction; RT-PCR, reverse transcriptase polymerase chain reaction.

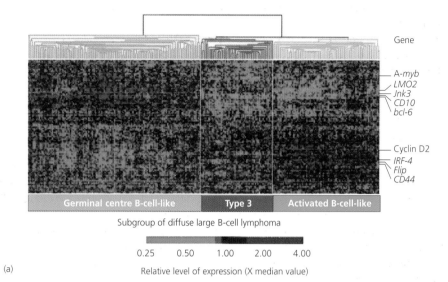

Subgroup of diffuse large B-cell lymphoma

Relative level of expression (X median value)

(a)

Oncogenic abnormality	Germinal centre B-cell-like	Type 3	Activated B-cell-like
		No. of samples	
c-rel amplification	17	0	0
bcl-2 t(14;18)	26	0	0

(b)

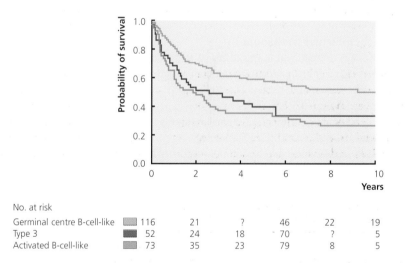

No. at risk

Germinal centre B-cell-like	116	21	?	46	22	19
Type 3	52	24	18	70	?	5
Activated B-cell-like	73	35	23	79	8	5

(c)

Figure 11.5 Gene expression profiling (GEP) of diffuse large B-cell lymphoma showing three patterns of expression that are associated with different clinical outcomes.

Treatment approaches: high grade malignancies

Approach for diffuse large B-cell lymphoma

Currently, in the UK, the gold standard treatment is CHOP (cyclophosphamide, doxorubicin, vincristine, and prednisone) chemotherapy with rituximab (see below). Issues that are currently in trial are the timing of chemotherapy (21-day versus 14-day cycle) and the number of cycles of treatment (six versus eight). Most patients (90%) will respond and about 50% of patients can be expected to be cured. The 10% who do not respond and the 40% who relapse should be treated with second line chemotherapy, with a view to high-dose therapy and a transplantation procedure if biologically fit and younger than 65 years. Elderly patients are potentially curable if biologically able to tolerate therapy, but their prognosis at relapse is poor.

Approach for mantle cell lymphoma

This is an aggressive lymphoma that appears incurable with currently available therapies. There is little evidence for superiority of intravenous over oral therapy, with both carrying a low complete remission rate. Some evidence supports consolidating a first response with a stem cell autologous transplant. Numerous experimental agents are currently in trial for this disease (for example, thalidomide, proteosome inhibitors such as bortezomib, and radiolabelled monoclonal antibodies).

Approach for Burkitt's lymphoma

This highly aggressive tumour, with a rapid doubling time (about 25 hours), requires treatment with brief duration, high-intensity chemotherapy regimens that contain aggressive CNS prophylaxis/treatment (see p. 65). In this setting, complete response rates are high (75–90%) and up to 80% of adults may be cured.

Approach for T-cell lymphomas

Although T-cell lymphomas include a spectrum of diverse pathological entities, they are in general clinically aggressive and more difficult to cure than B-cell malignancies. Initial treatment is often with CHOP chemotherapy. Transplantation should be considered, and trials of novel agents including monoclonal antibodies (Box 11.1) are important and ongoing.

Treatment approaches: low grade malignancies

The low grade malignancies tend to be indolent and may not require immediate treatment. Although they respond well to therapy, they are usually incurable and have a relapsing and remitting course. It is important to be clear about the desired impact of treatment. In elderly patients, simple non-toxic therapy to partially debulk disease without achieving a complete remission may be adequate. In younger patients, more aggressive strategies with greater side effects to maximally debulk disease and optimize the duration of response are more acceptable. It is important to recognize transformation from low to higher grade disease, as this requires more aggressive therapy and in general heralds a poor prognosis.

Approach for follicular lymphoma

A broad approach to treatment in this disease is to divide patients into those with asymptomatic and those with symptomatic disease.

- Asymptomatic disease. Most often a 'watch and wait' strategy is appropriate, but this requires careful explanation to patients who often associate no treatment with a terminal prognosis.
- Symptomatic disease. Treatment approaches include the use of oral agents such as chlorambucil, combination chemotherapy regimens (either fludarabine-containing or CHOP-like regimens) and newer strategies such as the use of radioimmunotherapy (see p. 61). The choice of regimen depends on the overall performance status of the patient and on the depth of remission that is aimed for. The addition of rituximab to chemotherapy produces better depth of remission and duration of response. The role of maintenance rituximab following chemotherapy is under exploration in current clinical trials.
- Relapse. All patients with follicular lymphoma treated with conventional chemotherapy will eventually relapse. Some will transform to diffuse large B-cell lymphoma (DLBCL). Treatment approaches are similar to those above, and choices depend on factors such as length of remission, response to certain agents previously and performance status. Autologous transplantation may be indicated in this setting, but is not curative, and allogeneic transplantation is considered in some patients.

Approach to the treatment of chronic lymphocytic leukaemia

Many patients will never require treatment and there is no evidence that early treatment in an asymptomatic patient is beneficial. Indications for treatment include: marrow failure, bulky disease, 'B' symptoms, or a rapid lymphocyte doubling time.

The specific therapy chosen should depend on the aim of treatment.

- In younger patients and those fit for transplantation, the aim is usually to achieve a complete remission with chemotherapy. These patients can be treated with agents such as fludarabine and cyclophosphamide and then progress to high-dose therapy and transplantation. The addition of rituximab (see above) may be advantageous.
- In the majority of patients, such an aggressive approach will not be appropriate, and the aim of treatment should be symptom control. Chlorambucil is the most common agent used; it has a high response rate and can be given orally and on an outpatient basis. Fludarabine is an alternative agent and, on its own or combined with cyclophosphamide, appears to be more active than chlorambucil. Most patients will relapse following a period of remission. Depending on the length of remission, they could be treated with the same agent again (long remission) or switched to the alternative agent with or without other agents (for example, cyclophosphamide).

Hodgkin's lymphoma

HL is a tumour with a high rate of cure. More than 80% of patients presenting in all stages can be cured. A minority of patients with very localized disease are curable by radiotherapy. Combination chemotherapy is the treatment of choice for most patients. The standard of care for patients with early stage disease is ABVD (doxorubicin, bleomycin, vinblastine and dacarbazine) chemotherapy, usually between 2–4 cycles, and this may be combined with radiotherapy. This is usually involved-field radiotherapy and trials are ongoing to ascertain whether radiotherapy is necessary in all cases (for example, in the context of PET scanning, see p. 65).

In the UK, advanced stage disease is usually treated with eight cycles of ABVD chemotherapy; however, other chemotherapy regimens have been shown to be equally efficacious. The role of radiotherapy after chemotherapy is the subject of current debate balancing efficacy against long-term risks. In view of the high rate of cure in this disease in young patients, there is a high risk of long-term treatment-related problems. It is estimated that those with a long-term cure

---

Box 11.1 **Monoclonal antibodies**

Monoclonal antibodies (MAbs) are antibodies that are targeted against specific molecules on the cell surface, resulting in cell death/destruction. The use of MAbs has revolutionized the treatment for many patients with lymphoma. In many settings the overall response rates to treatment are better with the addition of a MAb. Rituximab (an anti-CD20 Ab) is currently the most commonly used MAb, and its efficacy has been confirmed in numerous trials. This agent is approved by the National Institute of Clinical Excellence in certain clinical situations, and applications are in place to increase the accepted indications for this and other MAbs. In addition, agents in trial include a MAb conjugated to another substance (for example, a radioisotope) in an attempt to increase the specificity and kill of malignant cells.

eventually have a greater risk of mortality from treatment side effects than from HL (see below).

Special situations
Acquired immunodeficiency syndrome-related lymphomas
Historically, the outcome in these patients was dismal. The subtypes of lymphoma tend to be more aggressive or unusual than in non-acquired immunodeficiency syndrome (AIDS)-related cases. In addition, patients are more immunosuppressed than other categories of patient, both before and during treatment. Since the advent of highly active anti-retroviral therapy combined with chemotherapy, the outcome in patients has improved significantly, both in treating the lymphoma and in preventing opportunistic infections.

Central nervous system-directed treatment
CNS therapy may be given either for established disease or for prophylaxis. This will usually include systemic therapy with CNS penetration and intrathecal chemotherapy. Patients at high risk of CNS disease include those with Burkitt's lymphoma, lymphoblastic lymphoma, AIDS-related lymphomas, and a subset of patients with DLBCL, for example, widely disseminated disease, high lactate dehydrogenase (LDH) and particular extranodal sites of lymphoma.

Transplantation
The use of both autologous and allogeneic transplantation has greatly increased in recent years. This is due in part to the increased safety of these procedures. This should be considered early in the management of appropriate patients, both in order for referral to a transplant centre to be undertaken as well as for consideration of the agents with which to treat the patient (for example, avoiding agents that may decrease the likelihood of successful harvesting of autologous stem cells at a later stage).

Supportive care
Both the underlying disease and the treatments render these patients at high risk for infections (including atypical infections). In many situations, the use of prophylactic antimicrobials will be appropriate. These patients should be regularly followed up in clinic. Blood and platelet transfusions may be required.

Emergencies and management/prevention
Any patient presenting with the following emergencies must be discussed with a specialist at the earliest possible time.

Neutropenia
Neutropenia (bone marrow suppression) usually occurs about 10 days after chemotherapy. Sepsis during this period may be rapidly fatal. Patients presenting with a fever after chemotherapy should be assessed urgently, discussed with a specialist and, usually, commenced on intravenous antibiotics in accordance with the unit's protocol.

Superior vena cava obstruction
Patients with large mediastinal tumours may present with upper airway obstruction, which may be rapidly progressive. This often occurs in young patients. Treatment is with high-dose intravenous steroids or radiotherapy and should be commenced immediately in those with life-threatening symptoms. Thrombosis can occur.

Tumour lysis syndrome
Tumour lysis syndrome (TLS) is a medical emergency with a high morbidity and mortality. It is diagnosed on the basis of clinical and laboratory features that occur because of metabolic derangements resulting from tumour breakdown. Clinical symptoms include oliguria, cramps, seizures, cardiac failure and arrhythmias. Laboratory features include hyperphosphataemia, hypocalcaemia, hyperkalaemia and hyperuricaemia. It usually follows after chemotherapy; however, it may occasionally be spontaneous in highly proliferative diseases.

The most important aspect of TLS is prevention. This includes:
- Recognizing those patients at high risk (tumours with high proliferative rate, for example, Burkitt's lymphoma, lymphoblastic lymphoma, massive disease bulk, raised LDH, renal impairment).
- Using suitable prophylactic strategies (all patients should be adequately hydrated before and during chemotherapy). Those at high risk should receive rasburicase (urate oxidase enzyme that results in rapid degradation of uric acid) as prophylaxis. Others should receive allopurinol.
- Monitoring patients for the early recognition of TLS (as this complication usually occurs early after the start of chemotherapy. Routine blood tests should be performed at set times after treatment. Patients should be clinically assessed, particularly for urine output.

Treatment should be prompt and multidisciplinary. Early symptoms and metabolic derangements must be treated promptly, but this condition is generally rapidly progressive and many patients will require dialysis. Involvement by the renal team should be encouraged at an early stage.

Late effects
General
As the cure rate for many of the lymphoproliferative disorders increases, long-term survivors become more common and attention must be paid to the prevention of (avoidable) treatment side effects. HL occurs predominantly in young patients and may be used as an example to illustrate these points (see below). Storage of sperm should always be discussed prior to commencing therapy.

Hodgkin's lymphoma
Patients cured from HL should be followed up long term in order to actively monitor for, recognize and treat early treatment-related problems.

Secondary malignancy
- Lung cancer is the most common, related to radiotherapy. Smoking should be actively discouraged.
- Breast cancer is most common in women treated before the age of 30 years. The risk is dependent on the dose of radiotherapy. Screening should be carried out in those at risk.
- Acute myeloid leukaemia is related to the use of alkylating agents.
- Other malignancies may occur.

Cardiac disease
- Three-fold increase in cardiac death.
- Heart failure can complicate anthracycline usage.

Lung damage

- Radiation and bleomycin can cause fibrosis.

Endocrine

- Hypothyroidism is common, especially in those with irradiation to the neck.
- Infertility is related to irradiation and/or chemotherapy. Many of the current treatment approaches are fertility sparing, but the opportunity to store pretreatment material should always be discussed and offered.

Psychological

- Support should be offered to all at diagnosis, during and after treatment. This is particularly important in young adults, in whom lymphoma is a common malignancy.

Further reading

Burton C, Ell P, Linch D. The role of PET imaging in lymphoma. *British Journal of Haematology* 2004; **126**: 772–84.

Feugier P, Van Hoof A, Sebban C *et al*. Long-term results of the R-CHOP study in the treatment of elderly patients with diffuse large B-cell lymphoma: a study by the Groupe d'Etude des Lymphomes de l'Adulte. *Journal of Clinical Oncology* 2005; **23**: 4117–26.

Jaffe ES, Harris NL, Stein H *et al*. (eds). Tumours of haematopoietic and lymphoid tissues. In: *WHO Classification of Tumours*. IARC Press, Lyon, 2001.

McMillan A. Central nervous system-directed preventative therapy in adults with lymphoma. *British Journal of Haematology* 2005; **131**: 13–21.

Rosenwald A, Wright G, Chan WC *et al*. The use of molecular profiling to predict survival after chemotherapy for diffuse large-B-cell lymphoma. *New England Journal of Medicine* 2002; **346**: 1937–47.

CHAPTER 12

Stem Cell Transplantation

Fiona Clark, Charles Craddock

OVERVIEW

- Stem cell transplantation permits delivery of myeloablative doses of chemoradiotherapy without the risk of permanent marrow aplasia
- The anti-leukaemic effect of allogeneic stem cell transplantation is augmented by a graft-versus-leukaemia effect mediated by the donor immune system
- There is an intimate relationship between the potency of the graft-versus-leukaemia effect and the presence and severity of acute and chronic graft-versus-host disease
- Haemopoietic stem cells can be harvested from bone marrow or, increasingly, the peripheral blood
- The enhanced anti-leukaemic effect of allogeneic stem cell transplantation must be weighed against the risk of immediate and long-term complications of the procedure
- The use of reduced intensity conditioning regimens reduces the toxicity of allogeneic transplantation, permitting the extension of its potentially curative potential to older patients in whom transplantation has previously been contraindicated

Introduction

In the 1950s, it was shown in both animal models and humans that successful engraftment and haemopoietic recovery were achievable following infusion of bone marrow cells into lethally irradiated recipients. Over subsequent years, the discovery of histocompatibility antigens and improvements in tissue typing and supportive care led to the development of haemopoietic stem cell transplantation (HSCT) as a treatment for high risk haemopoietic malignancies and non-malignant bone marrow failure syndromes (Table 12.1).

The curative potential of HSCT lies firstly with the intensity of myeloablative chemoradiotherapy used to condition the recipient (the primary effector mechanism applied by autologous HSCT), and secondly with the ability of an allogeneic stem cell graft to mediate an immune effect against residual malignant cells, a property termed the graft-versus-leukaemia (GVL) effect. Reducing the intensity of the conditioning regimen in the allogeneic context (non-myeloablative conditioning) and the development of immune strategies to promote GVL have expanded the applicability of SCT to older patients in recent years.

Table 12.1 Current practice and indication for allogeneic and autologous transplantation in adults

	Autologous SCT	Allogeneic SCT	
		Sibling Tx	VUD Tx
AML 1st CR			
Good risk cytogenetics	NR	NR	NR
Standard risk cytogenetics	R	R	NR
Poor risk cytogenetics	R	R	R
AML 2nd CR	R	R	R
ALL 1st CR (normal cytogenetics)	D	R	NR
ALL 1st CR (t9;22)	R	R	R
ALL 2nd CR	R	R	R
CML 1st CP	NR	R	R
			(after trial of imatinib)
MDS	NR	R	R
Myeloma	R	R	D
Hodgkin's disease 1st CR	NR	NR	NR
Hodgkin's disease relapsed	R	D	D
NHL DLBCL 1st CR	D	NR	NR
NHL DLBCL relapse	R	D	D
NHL follicular relapse	R	R	D
Aplastic anaemia	NR	R	D
Haemoglobinopathies	NR	R	D

ALL, acute lymphoblastic leukaemia; MDS, myelodysplastic syndrome; AML, acute myeloid leukaemia; CML, chronic myeloid leukaemia; D, developmental; DLBCL, diffuse large B-cell lymphoma; NHL, non-Hodgkin's lymphoma; NR, not recommended; R, recommended.

Types of transplant (source of stem cells)

- Autologous (self).
- Syngeneic (identical twin donor).
- Human leucocyte antigen (HLA) matched sibling.
- HLA matched family member.
- HLA matched unrelated donor.
- HLA antigen mismatched donor.
- Haploidentical donor (HLA haplotype matched).
- Umbilical cord blood donor.

Haemopoietic stem cells

Haemopoietic stem cells (HSC) are long-term reconstituting cells that are defined by their dual ability to differentiate into all cells of the haemopoietic lineage, and to self renew. These cells normally reside in the bone marrow and circulate in the peripheral blood at extremely low frequency. In mouse models, HSC permit the repopulation of the marrow following myeloablative radiation. CD34, a cell surface glycoprotein expressed on early haemopoietic progenitors, is used as a marker of stem cells to aid collection and enumeration.

Following HSCT, engraftment and recovery of peripheral blood counts depend critically on the dose of HSC infused (expressed usually as CD34+ cells/kg body weight of the recipient). Cell dose predicts for speed of blood count recovery, immune reconstitution and transplant outcome. Engraftment following allogeneic transplantation also depends on important immune responses, which may be bidirectional (Fig. 12.1). Host-versus-graft immune responses, where recipient immunity is directed against components of the donor graft, may cause rejection of donor stem cells and is prevented by immune suppression of the recipient during preparative conditioning chemotherapy. Conversely, a graft-versus-host (GVH) reaction is mediated by the presence of donor T cells and natural killer cells in the graft, and recognizes recipient antigen mismatches. A GVH reaction has three key effects following allogenic transplantation: (i) facilitation of engraftment by depleting recipient residual immune cells; (ii) the development of acute and chronic graft versus host disease (GVHD); and (iii) mediated through a GVL effect, anti-tumour immunity.

HSC for transplantation can be obtained by two different techniques. Bone marrow may be aspirated from bilateral posterior iliac crests of the pelvis under general anaesthetic. A volume of marrow up to 1 L may be aspirated, with the aim of achieving a minimum cell dose based on recipient body weight that will reliably predict for engraftment. In recent years, the preferred collection technique mobilizes HSC into the peripheral blood using growth factor injections,

which are subsequently collected by leukapheresis. Granulocyte colony-stimulating factor (G-CSF) is administered to the donor by subcutaneous injection. High-dose G-CSF raises the peripheral blood white cell count and causes CD34+ stem cells to migrate from the marrow to circulate in the peripheral blood. After 4 or 5 days of G-CSF, the donor undergoes a leukapheresis procedure to collect the white cell fraction enriched for CD34+ stem cells. Compared with bone marrow as a graft, peripheral blood stem cells (PBSCs) provide faster blood count recovery and better immune reconstitution post-transplant. PBSC collection is a day-case procedure, avoids anaesthesia and there is no evidence of long-term effects from G-CSF administration to healthy volunteer donors. Common side effects include myalgia, bone pain and headache, and 2–5% of donors may go on to require a bone marrow harvest if insufficient cells are collected. This technique is increasingly being applied for autologous and allogeneic stem cell procurement, and donors are carefully counselled about both techniques.

Manipulation of a stem cell product may be performed in the allogeneic setting to deplete the graft of donor T cells and reduce the risk of GVHD. Techniques for this include:
- Immunomagnetic T-cell depletion.
- Immunomagnetic CD34+ cell selection.
- *In vitro* antibody depletion, for example the anti-CD52 antibody alemtuzumab (CamPath®; Genzyme).
- *In vivo* T-cell depletion with alemtuzumab or anti-thymocyte globulin.

Manipulation of an autologous stem cell product has been used in an attempt to reduce contaminating tumour cells, termed purging. For example, B-cell depletion for a B-cell lymphoma patient or CD34+ cell selection to give purified stem cells only.

Autologous stem cell transplantation

Autologous transplantation uses the patient's own blood stem cells as the graft and is the most common type of HSC transplant performed. Myelosuppression is the dose-limiting toxicity of chemotherapy, and at higher doses is associated with prolonged neutropenia, blood product requirement and risk of infection. The principle of autologous transplantation is to permit the safe delivery of high-dose chemotherapy followed by infusion of cryopreserved autologous stem cells, which allows blood count recovery after 2–3 weeks of predictable pancytopenia. This permits dose intensification of treatment and is used predominantly for patients with relapsed disease and high risk malignancy. Limitations to autologous transplant include the age and performance status of the patient and the ability to mobilize and collect sufficient HSC prior to transplant. Autologous HSCT is generally available to patients aged < 65–70 years with good performance status.

Standard indications for autologous haemapoietic stem cell transplantation
- Multiple myeloma in first disease response.
- Relapsed chemosensitive aggressive non-Hodgkin's lymphoma.
- Relapsed/refractory Hodgkin's disease.
- Relapsed acute myeloid leukaemia.
- Neuroblastoma and germ cell tumour (certain stages).

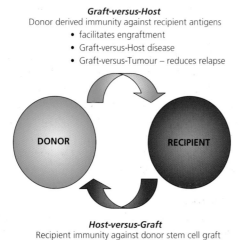

Graft-versus-Host
Donor derived immunity against recipient antigens
- facilitates engraftment
- Graft-versus-Host disease
- Graft-versus-Tumour – reduces relapse

DONOR   RECIPIENT

Host-versus-Graft
Recipient immunity against donor stem cell graft
- graft rejection

Figure 12.1 Immune responses following allogeneic stem cell transplantation are bidirectional.

Conditioning regimens in autologous stem cell transplantation

- High-dose melphalan ($200\,mg/m^2$) is the standard conditioning regimen in myeloma.
- BEAM [1,3-*bis*-(2-chloroethyl)-1-nitrosourea (BCNU; carmustine) $300\,mg/m^2$, etoposide $800\,mg/m^2$, cytosine arabinoside $800\,mg/m^2$ and melphalan $140\,mg/m^2$] is widely used in patients with lymphoma.
- Busulphan/cyclophosphamide and cyclophosphamide/total body irradiation (TBI) are myeloablative regimens effective for patients with acute leukaemia.
- Several other drug combinations incorporating melphalan, busulphan and thiotepa are used in solid tumours.

The transplant-related mortality (TRM) for autologous SCT is between 1 and 5% for most patients. Early effects and toxicities of autologous SCT predominantly reflect the acute effects of conditioning chemoradiotherapy (Box 12.1).

Late complications of autologous SCT include infertility, disease relapse and a small risk of secondary malignancy. Other late effects include pulmonary fibrosis in patients who have received BCNU or busulphan as part of their preparative regimen. TBI is associated with hypothyroidism and cataract formation, which may affect up to 10% of individuals.

Allogeneic stem cell transplantation

Immunology of allogeneic stem cell transplantation

The recent improvement in outcome following allogeneic transplantation is closely linked to a better understanding of the immunological basis that permits successful transplantation. An early key development was the understanding of the HLA system. An individual's HLA type is a set of highly polymorphic genes, expressed on the surface of cells. Disparity for these molecules between recipient and donor is known to predict for graft failure and GVHD and remains a major prognostic factor following transplant.

Allogeneic SCT is complicated by both the toxicities of preparative chemoradiotherapy, as outlined above (Box 12.1), and the immuno-logical reactions that can occur after transplant. Immune responses after transplant are bidirectional, occurring both as the host-versus-graft direction, where the recipient immune system recognizes donor antigens, and the GVH direction, where donor-derived immunity mounts a response against the recipient antigens (Fig. 12.1). An immune response in the host-versus-graft direction principally causes graft rejection and is reduced by immunosuppressive therapy during the conditioning regimen. Graft rejection is now rarely seen following fully HLA matched transplantation. The endpoints of a GVH immune response may be acute GVHD, chronic GVHD and anti-tumour immunity causing reduced risk of disease relapse (GVT).

Graft-versus-host disease

GVHD remains a major post-transplant complication, contributing significantly to transplant outcome, and may be acute or chronic in nature (Table 12.2). Acute GVHD commonly has its onset at or near the time of engraftment, and is defined as occurring < 100 days after transplant. It is characterized by a skin rash, liver function test abnormality and diarrhoea. The skin rash is maculopapular and is often limited to the palms and soles, responding to topical corticosteroids. Extensive rashes require systemic steroid therapy and in the worst case may progress to extensive erythroderma with bullae formation (Fig. 12.2). Liver GVHD causes rising bilirubin and alkaline phosphatase, and has characteristic histology with periportal lymphocytic infiltration and bile duct loss. Acute GVHD of the gastrointestinal tract presents with a secretory diarrhoea and/or abdominal pain. Severe disease is indicated by development of abdominal distension, ileus and pain with bloody diarrhoea. GVHD of the upper gut presents with anorexia, nausea and vomiting.

Chronic GVHD is the most common late complication of long-term survivors of allogeneic SCT. It is defined as occurring > 100 days after transplant and is a complex, often multisystem, disorder. Characteristic features include sclerodermatous skin changes, sicca syndrome, xerostomia, oesophageal stricture, malabsorption, contractures and bronchiolitis obliterans. Patients with extensive chronic GVHD require long-term immunosuppressive therapy, with ciclosporin and corticosteroids as the most common treatments. Infectious complications due to complex immune deficiency are frequent in this cohort and are the major cause of death.

Strategies to reduce GVHD include the administration of ciclosporin and methotrexate after transplant and T-cell depletion of the graft. Although highly effective at reducing the risk of severe acute GVHD, intensive T-cell depletion significantly affects immune reconstitution and, importantly, increases the risk of disease relapse by removing donor T cells that may mount a GVL response. The balance would ideally promote anti-tumour immunity without extensive severe GVHD, and this is the subject of current active research.

Donor selection

When searching for a donor for allogeneic transplant, initially HLA typing is performed for the recipient and available siblings. There is a one in four chance of siblings being matched for HLA class I and II molecules. Should a family member not be found, the next step is to consider a volunteer HLA matched unrelated donor search. The UK

Table 12.2 Clinical manifestations of acute and chronic graft-versus-host disease (GVHD)

Type	Appearance
Acute GVHD	
Skin	Limited/extensive maculopapular rash; generalized erythroderma, desquamation and bullae
Liver	Hyperbilirubinaemia and elevated alkaline phosphatase
Gut	Diarrhoea: may be high volume. Pain and ileus
Chronic GVHD	
Skin	Scleroderma, vitiligo, pigmentation, alopecia, nail dysplasia, contractures
Mucous membranes	Lichen planus, ulcers, corneal erosions, xerostomia, keratoconjunctivitis, sicca
Musculoskeletal	Myositis, arthritis, polyserositis, contractures
Lung	Bronchiolitis obliterans
Gut	Malabsorption, oesophageal strictures, diarrhoea, abdominal pain
Haematological	Thrombocytopenia, eosinophilia, autoantibodies and immune cytopenias
Liver	Elevated enzymes (alkaline phosphatase), cholangitis
Genitourinary	Vaginal stricture, vaginitis, atrophy

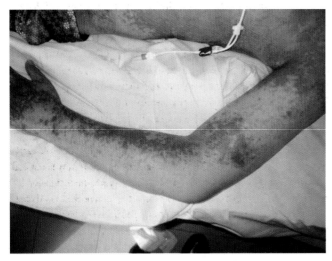

Figure 12.2 Skin involvement in graft-versus-host disease.

donor registries include the Anthony Nolan panel and the National Blood Service panel. Also available are international bone marrow donor registries. The chance of a successful unrelated donor search depends on HLA type and ethnicity, being highest for individuals of white northern European origin, who have a >60% chance of finding a matched donor. This reflects the predominant ethnicity of current donor panels. Improvement in outcome following unrelated donor transplantation is in part due to more detailed HLA matching at a molecular level and has reduced the mortality of unrelated donor transplantation over recent years.

Both sibling and unrelated donors are screened and must be assessed as medically fit prior to donation. They are now routinely offered either bone marrow harvest or G-CSF mobilized PBSC collection with leukapheresis. There is no evidence of any lasting adverse effects from G-CSF use in healthy donors, and therefore PBSCs are increasingly being used for both sibling and allogeneic SCT. Bone marrow and PBSC are significantly different in terms of cellular composition, with increased T-cell numbers in the PBSC graft. Despite this increase in donor T cells, interestingly there is no evidence

of increased acute GVHD or TRM with the use of PBSCs; however, chronic GVHD may be increased in long-term survivors.

Conditioning regimens

Preparative regimens for allogeneic transplantation previously entirely consisted of myeloablative conditioning regimes using protocols such as cyclophosphamide/TBI. The toxicity of these transplants excluded older patients and those with significant comorbidity from the curative potential of an allograft. The development of reduced intensity or non-myeloablative protocols in recent years has expanded the application of allogeneic transplantation and shows promising results (Box 12.2). Non-myeloablative regimens are more immunosuppressive than myelotoxic and allow the generation of stable mixed chimeras which can subsequently be converted to full donor chimeras. Consequently, these transplants rely predominantly on the genesis of a GVL effect immunity to control disease rather than the strength of conditioning regimen.

Infectious complications

In general, differing patterns of infectious complications are seen according to the time point after the allogeneic transplantation (Table 12.3). Early complications in the neutropenic period prior to engraftment include bacterial infections, viral infections such as cytomegalovirus (CMV) and fungal infections with *Candida* species

> **Box 12.2 Conditioning regimens in common UK practice for allogeneic stem cell transplantation**
>
> **Myeloablative**
> Cyclophosphamide 120 mg/kg, total body irradiation 12–14.4 Gy
> Cyclophosphamide 120 mg/kg, busulphan 14–16 mg/kg
> Melphalan 110 mg/kg, total body irradiation 12–14.4 Gy
>
> **Non-myeloablative**
> Fludarabine/melphalan/Campath 1H*
> BEAM (BCNU, etoposide, cytosine arabinoside, melphalan)/Campath 1H
>
> *Campath is a monoclonal antibody against CD52 surface protein; it depletes T cells and is broadly immunosuppressive

Table 12.3 Infectious complications following allogeneic stem cell transplant

Stage	Type of infection

Early (pre-engraftment)	Bacterial
	    Gram-positive and -negative
	Fungal
	    Candida
	    Aspergillus fumigatus
	Viral
	    Herpes simplex and zoster
	    Respiratory viruses

Intermediate (post-engraftment: 6 months)	Protozoal
	    Pneumocystis carinii
	    Toxoplasmosis
	Viral
	    Cytomegalovirus
	    Varicella zoster
	    Herpes simplex
	    Respiratory viruses

Late (long-term)	Bacterial
	    Encapsulated organisms
	    (*Streptococcus pneumoniae,*
	    Haemophilus influenzae)

and invasive *Aspergillus fumigatus*. Steps taken to reduce infection include patient isolation in rooms with filtered laminar-flow air, antifungal and antimicrobial prophylaxis, and prophylactic aciclovir to prevent herpes infection. Community respiratory viral pathogens, such as respiratory syncytial virus, influenza and parainfluenza, may be associated with significant risk of pneumonitis and secondary infection at early and intermediate stages after transplant.

Following engraftment, and for several months post-transplant, patients previously infected with CMV are at risk of virus reactivation, which occurs in 40–80% of at-risk individuals. CMV reactivation may be asymptomatic or progress to CMV disease, the most common manifestation of which is pneumonitis manifested by progressive dyspnoea and hypoxia. CMV disease may also cause gastrointestinal ulceration, hepatitis and retinitis. CMV was previously the commonest cause of infectious death after transplantation. Now, however, sensitive diagnostic tests may detect early viral reactivation in the blood and allow pre-emptive therapy with antiviral drugs. This improvement in supportive care has significantly reduced the incidence of CMV disease. Patients are also at risk of *Pneumocystis carinii* pneumonia (PCP) for several months until the cessation of immunosuppression, and therefore receive cotrimoxazole as proph-

ylaxis from the time of engraftment. Herpes zoster reactivation is seen in 40% of at-risk patients and may disseminate and rarely cause systemic and neurological infection.

Patients are advised to receive life-long penicillin V as prophylaxis against encapsulated organisms such as *Streptococcus pneumoniae* and *Haemophilus influenzae*, owing to functional hyposplenism, particularly following TBI-based regimens. At 12 months after transplant, patients are routinely fully revaccinated; of note, they must never receive live vaccines because of their impaired cellular immunity and risk of infection. Late infectious deaths are seen particularly in patients with chronic GVHD requiring immune suppression.

Conclusions and future developments

Autologous and allogeneic SCT remain the only curative therapies for many patients with high risk haematological malignancy and bone marrow failure syndromes. The application of allogeneic transplantation has been limited, firstly by the toxicity of conditioning regimens and secondly by the risk of severe GVHD or infectious complications. Reduced intensity transplantation employing less toxic and conditioning regimens has been a major development in allogeneic transplant practice and has expanded the cohort that may be eligible for these intensive therapies. Significant improvements in molecular techniques and HLA matching, supportive care strategies, and new antiviral and antifungal agents have all contributed to improved outcome for patients.

The challenge remains to further improve the safety and tolerability of these transplants. Key to this objective will be a more detailed understanding of the immunology that underpins these techniques and the development of immunotherapeutic strategies which can deliver tumour specific and pathogen specific cell therapy in the future.

Further reading

Bolanos-Meade J, Vogelsang GB. Acute graft-versus-host disease. *Clinical Advances in Clinical Hematology and Oncology* 2004; **2**: 672–82.

Craddock C, Chakraverty R. Stem cell transplantation. In: Hoffbrand AV, Catovsky D & Tuddenham E, eds. *Postgraduate Haematology*, 5th edn. 2005.

Gahrton G. Progress in hematopoietic stem cell transplantation in multiple myeloma. *Current Opinion in Hematology* 2005; **12**: 463–70.

Gratwohl A, Baldomero H, Schmid O *et al*. Change in stem cell source for hematopoietic stem cell transplantation (HSCT) in Europe: a report of the EBMT activity survey 2003.

Higman MA, Vogelsang GB. Chronic graft versus host disease. *British Journal of Haematology* 2004; **125**: 435–54.

Ljungman P, Urbano-Ispizua A, Cavazzana-Calvo M *et al*. Allogeneic and autologous transplantation for haematological diseases, solid tumours and immune disorders: definitions and current practice in Europe. *Bone Marrow Transplant* 2006; **37**: 439–49.

Peggs KS, Mackinnon S, Linch DC. The role of allogeneic transplantation in non-Hodgkin's lymphoma. *British Journal of Haematology* 2005; **128**: 153–68.

CHAPTER 13

Haematological Disorders at the Extremes of Life

Carolina Lahoz, Tyrell G J R Evans, Adrian C Newland

OVERVIEW

- Anaemia in the neonate results in reduced tissue oxygenation, metabolic acidosis and ultimately growth retardation and many other sequelae
- Neonatal thrombosis and thrombocytopenia are potentially lethal and prompt diagnosis and management are essential
- Elderly people are more susceptible to the effects of anaemia which is often multifactorial and should be investigated and treated appropriately
- The anaemia of chronic disease may be difficult to diagnose since it may mimic iron deficiency. This type of anaemia is not uncommon in the elderly and occurs in any chronic infective or inflammatory disorder, including cancer

Infants

Anaemia

The haemoglobin concentration at birth is 15.9–19.1 g/dL (Table 13.1). It rises transiently in the first 24 hours but then slowly falls to as low as 9.5 g/dL by 9 weeks. By 6 months, the concentration stabilizes at around 12.5 g/dL, the lower end of the adult range, increasing towards adolescence. The normal fall in haemoglobin concentration seen in full-term infants is accentuated in prematurity and may fall to <9.0 g/dL by 4 weeks. Preterm infants are particularly prone to multiple nutritional deficiencies because of rapid growth (Box 13.1).

Haemolytic disease of the fetus and newborn

Haemolytic disease of the fetus and newborn is caused by destruction of fetal red cells by antibodies (usually IgG) from the mother,

Table 13.1 Normal ranges for term and preterm infants

	Term	Preterm	Adult
Hb (g/dL)	14–24	14–24	11.5–18.0
Platelets (x 10⁹/L)	150–450	150–450	150–400
PT (s)	10–16	11–22	11–14
APTT (s)	31–55	31–101	27–40
TT (s)	19–28	19–30	12–14
Fibrinogen (g/L)	1.5–3.7	1.5–3.7	1.5–4

APTT, activated partial thromboplastin time; Hb, Haemoglobin; PT, prothrombin time; TT, thrombin time.

Box 13.1 **Common causes of anaemia in newborn infants**

- Blood loss: occult bleeding (fetomaternal, fetoplacental, twin to twin); obstetric accidents; internal bleeding; iatrogenic
- Increased destruction: immune haemolytic anaemia including haemolytic disease of the newborn; infection; haemoglobinopathies; enzymopathies
- Decreased production: infection; nutritional deficiencies, congenital syndromes

which cross the placenta. The most important are antibodies against the Rh (D) antigen. Maternal immunization is preventable by the prophylactic use of anti-D immunoglobulin, and since its introduction in 1969, the number of affected babies has fallen dramatically.

In severely affected fetuses, mortality used to be as high as 40%, with only exchange transfusion available after delivery to correct anaemia and prevent kernicterus. Intrauterine transfusion using fetoscopy into the umbilical artery has greatly improved survival. Hydrops can be readily reversed *in utero*, and even in the most severe group the survival rate is 85%.

Haemoglobinopathies
Thalassaemias

β Thalassaemia major is caused by reduction in β globin chain synthesis. It affects primarily people from the Indian subcontinent and of Mediterranean origin. It presents during the first year of life after the switch from fetal to adult haemoglobin. If production of the latter is reduced, anaemia occurs. The infant presents with failure to thrive, poor weight gain, feeding problems and irritability. The blood appearances are typical, with severe anaemia associated with microcytosis and hypochromia as well as pronounced morphological changes in the red cells. The infant will be dependent on transfusions unless bone marrow transplantation is feasible. The carrier state (thalassaemia minor or thalassaemia trait) mimics iron deficiency, from which it must be differentiated (Fig. 13.1, Table 13.2).

Sickle cell disease

Sickle cell disease is caused by a structural abnormality of the β globin chain and is associated with a steady-state haemoglobin of 5.0–11.0 g/dL (Box 13.2). In homozygous sickle cell disease, the haemoglobin is insoluble and forms crystals when exposed to low oxygen

Table 13.2 Features of α thalassaemia

Syndrome	Haematological abnormalities	Diagnosis
Silent carrier (–α/αα)*	No anaemia or microcytosis	1–2% Hb Bart's†
Thalassaemia trait (–α/–α)	Mild anaemia and microcytosis	3–10% Hb Bart's
Hb H disease (–/–α)	Moderate microcytic, hypochromic, haemolytic anaemia	20–40% Hb Bart's
Hb Bart's hydrops syndrome (– –/– –)	Severe microcytic, hypochromic anaemia (lethal)	80% Hb Bart's, 20% Hb H‡

*Where αα/αα is normal (that is, four α genes) and –α represents deletion of one α gene on a chromosome.
†Bart's γ_4 tetramers.
‡Hb H β_4 tetramers. Hb, haemoglobin.

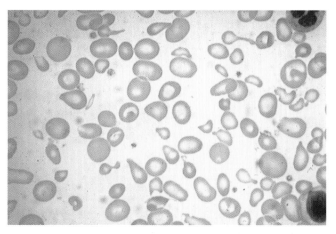

Figure 13.1 Peripheral blood of patient with haemoglobin H disease showing pale red cells (hypochromia) with variation in size and shape (anisopoikilocytosis).

tension, distorting the red blood cells into a rigid sickle cell shape. These sickle cells block the microvasculature, causing infarcts and leading to sickle cell crises. Mortality and morbidity are increased at all ages, with the peak incidence of death at the age of 1–3 years.

Enzyme deficiencies

Glucose-6-phosphate dehydrogenase deficiency and pyruvate kinase deficiency are the most common and can present in childhood. Haemolytic anaemia typically occurs under stress.

Box 13.2 Treatment for sickle cell disease

- Antenatal screening for carrier detection of sickle cell disease should be carried out in pregnant women and partners if indicated, so that genetic counselling and prenatal diagnosis can be offered
- Universal neonatal screening for sickle cell disease is being implemented in the UK. This programme will also detect most other haemoglobinopathies such as β thalassaemia
- Penicillin prophylaxis and an adequate vaccination programme are the main health procedures that have succeeded in prolonging survival, by reducing encapsulated organism infections
- Transfusion programmes for those with severe disease (chest crises, strokes) are expected to improve survival and quality of life

---

Membrane defects

Hereditary spherocytosis should be suspected if there is a family history and haemolysis. It is the commonest cause of inherited chronic haemolysis in northern Europe and North America.

Sepsis, bleeding, prematurity

Cytomegalovirus, rubella, toxoplasmosis, HIV (Box 13.3) and, more rarely, congenital syphilis may be associated with anaemia, due either to haemolysis or bone marrow suppression. More recently, human parvovirus B19 has been identified as a cause of anaemia and fetal damage. It may also induce an aplastic crisis or chronic haemolysis in normal children, but is a major problem in those with an underlying haemoglobinopathy.

Malaria is a major health hazard worldwide, and easier travel to endemic areas has increased the problem. Inadequate prophylaxis has led to an increase in cases over the past few years; unsuspected infection in neonates, usually caught from the mother, may be associated with a high mortality.

Iron deficiency anaemia

Anaemia affects more than 500 million people worldwide, most of them in developing countries, mainly women and infants.

Congenital bone marrow failure syndromes

Congenital bone marrow failure syndromes are usually apparent within the first years of life and present with other abnormalities (Table 13.3).

Bleeding and thrombotic disorders

Clotting factor deficiencies may present symptomatically in the

---

Box 13.3 Human immunodeficiency virus infection

- Human immunodeficiency virus (HIV) may produce a chronic multisystem disease in children
- Perinatal transmission of the virus from an infected woman is the primary route of exposure to the fetus (20–40% of pregnancies)
- Thrombocytopenia occurs in up to 15% of children with HIV infection
- Anaemia is also common, occurring early, usually with the normocytic, normochromic features of chronic disease
- Leucopenia and lymphopenia are also seen, in which the bone marrow shows non-specific features of chronic infection

Table 13.3 Features of Fanconi's anaemia and congenital dyskeratosis

Fanconi's anaemia	Congenital dyskeratosis
Autosomal recessive	X-linked recessive
Absent thumbs/radius, microcephaly, short stature	Skin pigmentation
Renal anomalies	Leukoplakia
Abnormal pigmentation	Dystrophic nails
High incidence of MDS/AML	

In up to 30% of all new cases, patients will have no family history of coagulation disorders, and such cases are therefore new mutations. AML, acute myeloid leukaemia; MDS, myelodysplastic syndrome.

Box 13.4 **Common causes of thrombocytopenia**

- Immune-mediated
  - Neonatal alloimmune thrombocytopenia
  - Maternal immune thrombocytopenic purpura
  - Drug-induced
- Infection
  - Viral, e.g. cytomegalovirus, human immunodeficiency virus, rubella
  - Toxoplasmosis
- Post-exchange transfusion
- Disorders of haemostasis
  - Disseminated intravascular coagulation
  - Maternal pre-eclampsia
  - Rhesus isoimmunization
  - Hypothermia, hypoxia
  - Type IIB von Willebrand's disease
- Liver disease
- Giant haemangioma
- Hereditary thrombocytopenia
- Marrow infiltration

---

first days of life, with spontaneous bleeding (Table 13.4). Severe bleeding usually occurs at circumcision or when mobility increases. Thrombosis may present in the neonatal period (Table 13.5).

Thrombocytopenia

Thrombocytopenia is the most common haemostatic abnormality in newborn infants, occurring in up to a quarter of babies admitted to neonatal intensive treatment units. Platelet transfusions should be given to any infant whose count is $< 20 \times 10^9$/L (Box 13.4).

Table 13.4 Haemorrhagic diseases of newborn infants

Possible deficiencies	Pattern	Treatment
Factor VIII	X-linked	Recombinant factor VIII
Factor IX	X-linked	Recombinant factor IX
von Willebrand factor	AR/AD	Desmopressin, plasma derived products
Vitamin K	Acquired, e.g. breastfed from mother on anticonvulsants or warfarin	Vitamin K, fresh frozen plasma

AD, autosomal dominant; AR, autosomal recessive.

Table 13.5 Neonatal thrombosis

Aetiology	Protein C deficiency	Sick, preterm infants
	Protein S deficiency	Inherited
Diagnosis	Doppler ultrasound. Contrast angiography	
Management	Supportive care. Anticoagulant therapy with heparin. Thrombolytic therapy and surgery, which should take place in a specialized centre. Protein C concentrate is available and fresh frozen plasma can be given for replacement of protein S	

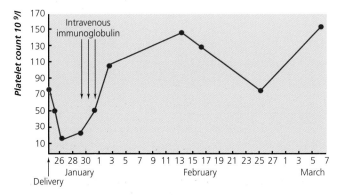

Figure 13.2 Response of neonate with thrombocytopenia secondary to maternal immune thrombocytopenic purpura to intravenous immunoglobulin. Copyright ©1984 Massachusetts Medical Society. All rights reserved. Adapted with permission from Newland et al. *New England Journal of Medicine* 1984; **310**: 261–2.

Maternal autoimmune thrombocytopenia may be associated with neonatal thrombocytopenia because of placental transfer of antiplatelet antibodies. Fetal platelet counts rarely drop below 50×10^9/L, but the count may fall in the first few days of life, and treatment may be needed at this stage.

There are no reliable predictors of severe thrombocytopenia. Treatment includes platelet transfusions and corticosteroids, but intravenous immunoglobulin is safe and effective in over 80% of infants (Fig. 13.2).

Neonatal alloimmune thrombocytopenia

This condition affects 1 in 2000 live births and accounts for 10% of all cases of neonatal thrombocytopenia. Maternal platelet counts are

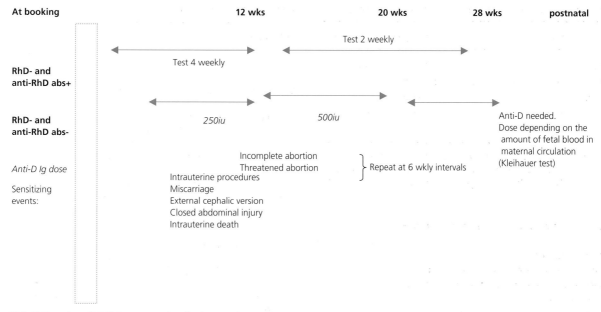

Figure 13.3 RhD testing: ABO RhD group and antibody screening.

normal, and maternal alloantibodies are directed against paternally derived antigens on the infant's platelets [usually human platelet antigen (HPA)-1]. Clinical manifestations of neonatal alloimmune thrombocytopenia (NAIT) vary from mild (petechiae and bruises) to severe (intracranial haemorrhage with possible death or life-long morbidity). NAIT is associated with severe thrombocytopenia, and intracranial haemorrhage is seen in up to 15% of infants. In at-risk pregnancies, fetal blood sampling by cordocentesis should be used to confirm the HPA-1 status. Treatment consists of platelet transfusions *in utero*, but high-dose intravenous immunoglobulin may be of some benefit.

The firstborn is affected in 40–60% of cases, and the condition is usually unexpected. Subsequent pregnancies are affected in 75–90% of cases with similar or increasing severity. Intrauterine death occurs in up to 10% of cases.

Transfusion in the fetus, neonate and older infant

Packed red cells are given *intra utero* to treat red cell alloimmunization (haemolytic disease of the newborn) and parvovirus-induced anaemia. Neonatal exchange transfusion will be required if there is severe anaemia (and the volume of red cells may cause fluid overload), or to treat hyperbilirubinaemia. Children with β thalassaemia major or those with sickle cell anaemia who have suffered strokes will need long-term transfusions. Hepatitis B vaccination is required, and iron chelation will be needed after 10 transfusions or when ferritin is higher than 1000 μg/L.

Intrauterine platelet transfusions are used to prevent NAIT and this is carried out in specialized centres.

Fresh frozen plasma in the UK is imported from countries with a low incidence of bovine spongiform encephalopathy and treated with methylene blue for all children born after 1 January 1996.

This population has very specific transfusion requirements and guidelines have been drawn up by the British Committee for Standards in Haematology (BCSH) (Box 13.5).

Box 13.5 BCSH Guidelines

- Donors for children < 1 year of age must have donated at least once within the past 2 years
- Leucocyte depletion of blood products
- Cytomegalovirus (CMV): in the first year of life the blood should be CMV seronegative
- Irradiation: intrauterine transfusions (IUT), exchange transfusions after IUT, donations from first- or second-degree relative or human leucocyte antigen-matched donor, recipient diagnosed with immunodeficiency, children undergoing transplant or receiving fludarabine must be irradiated to a minimum dose of 25 Gy
- Plasma and platelet compatibility: platelets should be ABO and Rh(D) identical with the recipient
- All components should be transfused through an administration set with a screen filter

---

Neutropenia

Sepsis is the most common cause of neutropenia but neonatal alloimmune neutropenia and racial neutropenia, familial chronic benign neutropenia and the rarer congenital conditions, such as Schwachmann's syndrome and reticular dysgenesis, must be considered.

Polycythaemia

Defined as a venous haematocrit of > 65%, polycythaemia is a relatively common disorder. The primary concern with polycythaemia is related to hyperviscosity and its associated complications.

Polycythaemia occurs in 0.4–12% of neonates and is more common in infants who are small or large for their gestational age. Infants of mothers with diabetes have a > 40% incidence of polycythaemia, and those born to mothers with gestational diabetes have an incidence exceeding 30%. Hyperviscosity occurs in 6.7% of infants.

Table 13.6 Adverse prognostic factors in acute leukaemia

Adverse risk factors	Symptoms
White cell count	Fever (60%)
Age	Fatigue (50%)
Translocations	Pallor (25%)
Hypodiploidy	Weight loss (26%)
Slow early response	Bone pain (23%)
	CNS involvement (5%)

CNS, central nervous system.

Leukaemia

Acute lymphoblastic leukaemia is the most common form of leukaemia in children. Children develop symptoms related to infiltration of malignant lymphoblasts in the bone marrow, lymphoid system and extramedullary sites, and disruption of normal haemopoiesis. Complete remission is achieved in 98% and long-term disease survival is 70–75%. Treatment consists of several phases (induction, consolidation, central nervous system prophylaxis and maintenance). High risk children and those who relapse are offered allogeneic bone marrow transplantation from matched sibling or unrelated (including cord) donors (Table 13.6).

Elderly people

The haemoglobin concentration gradually declines from the age of 60 years, with a more rapid fall over the age of 70 years. The fall is accompanied, however, by a widening of the reference range, thus age-dependent ranges are of little value in individuals. The haemoglobin concentration should be considered in association with the clinical history. In older patients the lower end of the normal range should be reduced to 11.0 g/dL.

Iron deficiency anaemias

Between 10 and 20% of elderly people will be anaemic, usually with iron deficiency (Box 13.6). In many, this will be nutritional, owing to difficulties in obtaining and eating food, for both medical and social reasons. The possibility of an occult gastrointestinal malignancy (for example, caecal carcinoma) leading to iron deficiency anaemia should be considered. Aspirin or non-steroidal anti-inflammatory drugs leading to occult gastrointestinal blood loss may also contribute. The problem may also be exacerbated in elderly people as gastric atrophy may occur, leading to poor absorption of iron supplements.

> ### Box 13.6 Clinical associations in iron deficiency
>
> - Symptoms: lethargy, lassitude, reduced activity; shortness of breath; angina on effort; intermittent claudication
> - Signs: pallor, peripheral oedema; brittle nails, koilonychia; glossitis; stomatitis
> - Other gastrointestinal findings: oesophageal web; atrophic gastritis; subtotal villous atrophy with malabsorption

---

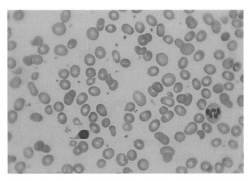

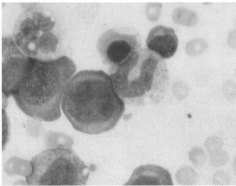

Figure 13.4 Megaloblastic anaemia: peripheral blood (top) showing macrocytes, tear drops, and multisegmented neutrophils; megaloblastic bone marrow (bottom) showing megaloblasts, giant metamyelocytes, and hypersegmented neutrophil.

Oral supplements are usually well tolerated. They should be continued for 3 months after the haemoglobin concentration has returned to normal, to replenish the iron stores.

Megaloblastic anaemia

Folic acid deficiency also occurs readily in those who eat poorly and can be easily corrected by supplements. Pernicious anaemia due to vitamin B_{12} deficiency also occurs in middle and later life, and may be associated with weakness and loss of sensation. Vitamin B_{12} stores normally fall in older people, and deficiency should always be considered with those developing dementia.

Care must be taken to differentiate megaloblastic anaemia from myelodysplastic syndrome (Fig. 13.4), which may be associated with a refractory macrocytic anaemia. Serum concentrations of vitamin B_{12}, folate and red cell folate should be measured, and occasionally a bone marrow examination may be indicated.

The deficiencies can be easily reversed, and supplements should be continued for as long as the underlying problem remains.

Anaemia of chronic disease

Any prolonged illness such as infection, malignant disease, renal disease, or connective tissue disorder may be accompanied by a moderate fall in the haemoglobin concentration (Box 13.7). This seldom drops below 9.0–10.0 g/dL, and is typically normocytic and normochromic. Supplements will not increase the haemoglobin concentration, which may improve only after treatment of the underlying condition. This condition may not always be apparent, and a general screen may be needed for underlying malignancy or systemic disease (Box 13.8).

Malignancies

Most forms of malignancy are more common in elderly people than in the rest of the population. The myelodysplastic syndromes and chronic lymphocytic leukaemia are frequently found incidentally, and their diagnosis does not necessarily indicate the need for treatment. Each patient must be considered individually so that the possible benefits of treatment can be balanced against side effects and considered in the light of any improvement in the quality of life. Ongoing therapeutic trials should be considered when appropriate.

Further reading

Bolton-Maggs PH, Stevens RF, Dodd NJ *et al.* Guidelines for the diagnosis and management of hereditary spherocytosis. *British Journal of Haematology* 2004; **126:** 455–74.

Gibson BE, Todd A, Roberts I *et al.* Transfusion guidelines for neonates and older children. *British Journal of Haematology* 2004; **124:** 433–53.

Guralnik JM, Ershler WB, Schrier SL *et al.* Anemia in the elderly: a public health crisis in hematology. *Hematology. American Society of Hematology Educational Program* 2005: 528–32.

Hann IM, Gibson BES, Letsky EA, eds. *Fetal and Neonatal Haematology.* Baillière Tindall, London, 1991.

Lilleyman JS, Hann IM, eds. *Pediatric Hematology*, 2nd edn. Churchill Livingstone, New York, 1999.

O'Shaughnessy DF, Atterbury C, Bolton Maggs P *et al.* Guidelines for the use of fresh-frozen plasma, cryoprecipitate and cryosupernatant. *British Journal of Haematology* 2004; **126:** 11–28.

Public Health Service Task Force. *Interventions to Reduce Perinatal HIV-1 Transmission in the US.* 17 November, 2005.

Spiers ASD. Management of the chronic leukemias: special considerations in the elderly patient. Part 1. Chronic lymphocytic leukemias. *Hematology* 2001; **6:** 291–314.

CHAPTER 14

Haematological Emergencies

Jim Murray, Belinda Austen, Drew Provan

OVERVIEW

- Haematological emergencies require prompt recognition for prompt treatment
- Spinal cord compression may be the presenting feature in myeloma
- Platelet transfusions may be lifesaving in disseminated intravascular coagulation
- Platelet transfusions should be avoided in thrombotic thrombocytopenic purpura
- Accurate diagnosis of TTP is crucial to ensure appropriate management

The importance of the prompt treatment of severe neutropenic sepsis in patients receiving chemotherapy for the treatment of malignant disease is now well recognized. Life-threatening complications such as disseminated intravascular coagulation or spinal cord compression may present to the general physician in a variety of clinical circumstances, and prompt recognition of the underlying pathology is crucial for successful management.

Hyperviscosity syndrome

This may result from a number of haematological conditions (Box 14.1). Whole blood viscosity is a function of the concentration and composition of its components, but is also very dependent upon flow rates. Blood viscosity will be increased by an elevation in the cellular constituents (Fig. 14.1) (for example, white blood cells in acute leukaemia and red cells in polycythaemia) or by an increase in plasma proteins (for example, a monoclonal immunoglobulin in myeloma or lymphoma). The higher viscosity in small vessels leads to sluggish capillary blood flow, which is responsible for the clinical features.

Box 14.1 Causes of hyperviscosity

- Waldenström's macroglobulinaemia
- Acute leukaemia with hyperleucocytosis (high white cell count)
- Polycythaemia vera
- Myeloma

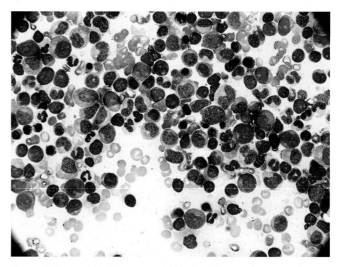

Figure 14.1 Blood film in acute myeloid leukaemia. Note the extremely high number of circulating white blood cells (hyperleucocytosis), leading to hyperviscosity.

Signs and symptoms of hyperviscosity include neurological disturbance, retinopathy (Fig. 14.2) and spontaneous bleeding, usually epistaxis (Table 14.1). The severity of the clinical picture will depend on the characteristics of the cell type or protein that is increased, and

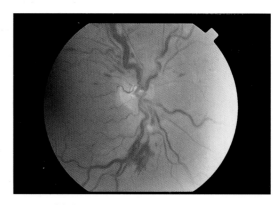

Figure 14.2 Fundal changes in a patient with hyperviscosity (newly diagnosed myeloma) with IgA concentration 50 g/dL.

Table 14.1 Symptoms and signs of hyperviscosity

Symptom	Sign
Headache	
Neurological disturbance	Changes in mental state
	Confusion
	Coma
Ocular disturbance	Dilatation and segmentation of retinal veins
Bleeding	Epistaxis

will also reflect the level of physiological compensation. Patients with chronic disorders such as polycythaemia vera often only complain of mild headaches, whereas patients with acute leukaemia, notably acute myeloid leukaemias, may present *in extremis*, with marked hypoxia from pulmonary leucostasis, together with altered consciousness and a variety of neurological signs related to reduced cerebral blood flow. Hyperviscosity may also precipitate cardiac failure in susceptible patients.

The definitive management of hyperviscosity is through treatment of the underlying condition, usually with chemotherapy. Prompt treatment is needed in severe cases to prevent permanent deficits. For patients presenting with acute leukaemias, leukapheresis may be used as an interim measure until the chemotherapy exerts its full effect. Vigorous hydration and uricosuric agents (rasburicase) are also indicated. For patients with hyperviscosity due to elevated immunoglobulins (often IgM or IgA), plasmapheresis is effective in reducing the paraprotein concentration. This may be necessary at disease presentation, but can also be performed at regular intervals in symptomatic patients with chemotherapy refractory disease. For patients with polycythaemia, isovolaemic venesection will reduce the blood viscosity.

Sickle cell crisis

The sickling disorders result from the inheritance of structural haemoglobin (Hb) variants. Homozygous sickle cell anaemia (Hb SS) is the most common and severe form of sickle cell anaemia in the UK. The compound heterozygotes comprising Hb S in association with Hb C (Hb SC), β thalassaemia (Hb S/β thal) or Hb D (Hb SD) account for the majority of the remaining cases.

Recurrent episodes of acute, severe pain due to vaso-occlusive sickle cell crises are the hallmark of these diseases (Table 14.2). Crises can also result from marrow aplasia, splenic or hepatic sequestration and episodes of haemolysis. The chest syndrome and the girdle syndrome are more severe forms of crisis associated with higher morbidity and mortality (Fig. 14.3). Other complications include leg ulcers, renal impairment and retinopathy (Hb SS), and thrombosis (Hb SC).

Dehydration, infection, stress or skin cooling may precipitate vaso-occlusive crises. Sickling of the red cells occurs in the small vessels resulting in decreased tissue blood flow and hypoxia and acidosis, which in turn precipitate further sickling (Fig. 14.4).

The aim of treatment is to break this cycle of sickling (Box 14.2). Management, therefore, includes the maintenance of a high fluid intake (60 mL/kg/24 h) to prevent dehydration and oxygen therapy if hypoxia is confirmed on pulse oximetry. Imperative to the management of patients with sickle cell crises is adequate pain relief. This often requires opiates, given as continuous intravenous or subcutaneous infusions. Sickle cell patients are functionally asplenic, and broad spectrum antibiotics should be started in any patient in whom infection is suspected.

Top-up blood transfusions are often unnecessary and should be reserved for patients with signs or symptoms attributable to anaemia, typically when the Hb has fallen more than 2 g/dL and is <5 g/dL. Transfused red cell products should be matched for Rh (C, D and E) and Kell antigens. Exchange transfusions aim to reduce the level of Hb S to <30% and are indicated in patients with severe chest syndrome, suspected cerebrovascular events, priapism or multiorgan failure. Any patient requiring an exchange transfusion should be discussed with a haematologist.

Spinal cord compression

Patients with haematological disease may present with spinal cord compression. This may be due to tumour deposits, such as lym-

Table 14.2 Sickle cell crises

Type	Affected area/causes	Symptoms
Commonly		
Vaso-occlusive: can affect any tissue	Bones	Dactylitis
	Abdomen	Splenic infarcts
	Brain	Cerebral infarcts
	Chest	Pleuritic pain, may develop into 'chest syndrome', which is associated with progressive respiratory failure
Rarely		
Aplastic	Due to parvovirus B19 infection	
Sequestration	Due to pooling of red cells in spleen or other organs	
Haemolytic	Due to a further reduction in the red cell lifespan	

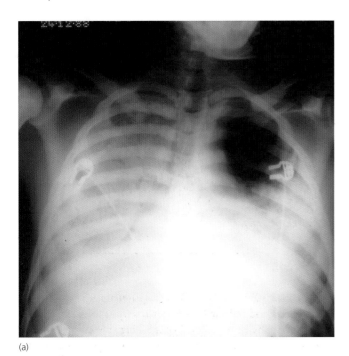

(a)

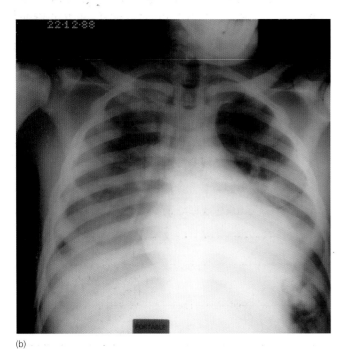

(b)

Figure 14.3 Sickle cell disease. (a) AP chest radiograph before treatment shows generalized air space change/consolidation throughout the right lung and in the left lower zone. (b) AP chest radiograph post-treatment showing improved aeration bilaterally with some resolution of the bilateral air space changes.

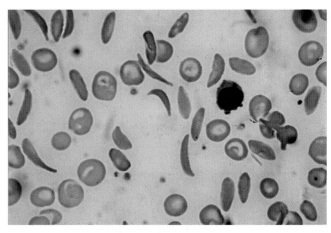

Figure 14.4 Sickled red cells (crescent-shaped) in homozygous sickle cell disease.

Box 14.2 **Treatment of sickle cell crises**

Adequate analgesia: usually will require opiates
- Vigorous intravenous hydration
- Oxygen: if hypoxia
- Broad spectrum antibiotics: if signs of infection
- Consider top-up transfusions if Hb has fallen > 2 g/dL
- Consider exchange transfusion for the chest syndrome, stroke or multiorgan failure

---

The neurological signs accompanying cord compression vary according to both the rapidity of the development of compression and the area of the cord affected (Box 14.3). Acute lesions often result in hypotonia and weakness, whereas chronic lesions are more often associated with the classic upper motor neurone signs of hypertonia and hyper-reflexia. The site of the lesion defines the associated sensory loss, and hyperaesthesia may be seen in the dermatome at the level of the lesion. More lateral lesions may result in dissociated sensory loss, that is, ipsilateral loss of joint position sense, and proprioception with contralateral loss of pain and temperature. Bladder and bowel disturbances often occur late, with the exception of the cauda equina compression syndrome, in which they are an early feature.

If cord compression is suspected, the definitive investigation is an urgent magnetic resonance scan (Fig. 14.5) to establish the presence of cord compression, to delineate the level of the lesion and to plan further treatment. Plain spinal X-rays are useful if myeloma is suspected to demonstrate lytic lesions.

In the acute presentation, high-dose dexamethasone, for example, 4 mg four times daily, is given. In a patient presenting *de novo*

phoma or plasmacytoma, or a consequence of spinal instability from lytic bone disease in multiple myeloma. Most patients with cord compression complain of pain, which is constant and can be easily confused with degenerative disease. Commonly, signs consistent with root compression, with pain in the affected dermatome, precede the overt signs of cord compression.

Box 14.3 **Symptoms and signs of cord compression**

- Back pain
- Leg weakness
- Upper motor neurone and sensory signs
- Loss of sphincter control (bowels and bladder)

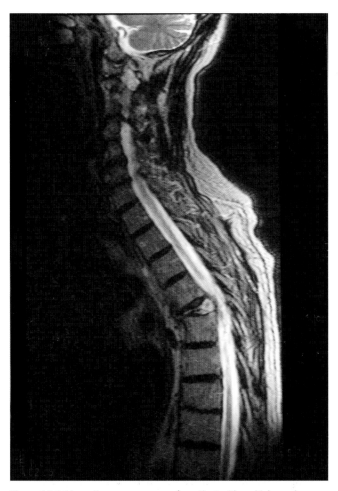

Figure 14.5 Magnetic resonance scan of a patient with multiple myeloma showing complete collapse of T5 vertebra with an acquired short segment kyphosis and spinal cord compression.

with cord compression, investigations are aimed at establishing an underlying diagnosis, and will usually include protein electrophoresis, measurement of tumour markers including prostate specific antigen, imaging such as a chest X-ray and/or computed tomography scans, and a tissue biopsy of the lesion to establish the histology. Further management will then depend on the underlying cause, and will often involve a combination of chemotherapy and radiotherapy.

Disseminated intravascular coagulation

Disseminated intravascular coagulation (DIC) describes the syndrome of widespread intravascular coagulation induced by blood procoagulants either introduced into or produced in the bloodstream (Table 14.3). These coagulant proteins overcome the normal physiological anticoagulant mechanisms. The overall result, irrespective of the cause, is widespread tissue ischaemia (due to clot formation, thrombi) and bleeding (due to consumption of clotting factors, platelets, and the production of breakdown products that further inhibit the coagulation pathway).

If the diagnosis of DIC is suspected clinically, investigations should include a full blood count, clotting profile, fibrinogen level

Table 14.3 Clinical features of disseminated intravascular coagulation

Disorder	Features
Bleeding	Spontaneous bruising and petechiae
	Prolonged bleeding from venepuncture sites
	Epistaxis
	Gastrointestinal bleeding
	Pulmonary haemorrhage
	Intracerebral bleed
Thrombosis	Venous thromboembolism
	Skin necrosis
	Acute renal failure (ischaemia of the renal cortex)
	Cerebral infarction
Features related to the underlying disorder	Shock

and D-dimers (Table 14.4). In DIC, the platelet count is decreased, prothrombin and activated partial thromboplastin times elevated, fibrinogen level decreased and D-dimers increased.

Treatment is primarily directed at the underlying cause (Table 14.5), for example, antibiotics for infection, the removal of the fetus or placenta in cases of retained dead fetus syndrome or placental abruption, or treatment with chemotherapy for acute promyelocytic leukaemia. DIC generally resolves fairly quickly after removal of the underlying cause in obstetric cases, but control of septicaemia can take some time.

Interim supportive measures include intravenous hydration, oxygen therapy and correction of the coagulopathy. Platelet transfusions are generally indicated when the count is $< 50 \times 10^9/L$, fresh frozen plasma to replace clotting factors when the international normalized ratio or activated partial thrombin ratio is > 1.5, and cryoprecipitate when the fibrinogen level is $< 1.0\,g/L$ (Box 14.4). The use of intrave-

Table 14.4 Essential diagnostic investigations for disseminated intravascular coagulation

Investigation	Positive result
Full blood count	Reduced platelet count
Prothrombin time	Increased
Activated partial thromboplastin time	Increased
Fibrinogen	Decreased
D-dimers	Increased

Table 14.5 Causes of acute disseminated intravascular coagulation

Type	Cause
Infection	Gram-negative infections, endotoxic shock
Obstetric	Placental abruption, intra-uterine death, severe pre-eclampsia or eclampsia, amniotic fluid embolism
Trauma	Head injury, burns
Malignancy	Carcinoma of the prostate, ovary, colon, pancreas. Acute promyelocytic leukaemia
Vascular	Aortic aneurysm, giant haemangioma
Miscellaneous	Transfusion with ABO incompatible blood, hypothermia, drug reactions

Box 14.4 **Initial management of disseminated intravascular coagulation**

- Treat as for severe bleeding/shock
- Administer platelets, if platelet count < 50×10⁹/L
- Administer fresh frozen plasma to correct prothrombin time and activated partial thromboplastin time
- Administer cryoprecipitate, if fibrinogen is < 1.0 g/L
- Remove/treat the underlying cause

Table 14.6 Clinical subtypes of thrombotic thrombocytopenic purpura (TTP)

Type	Subtype	Cause
Congenital		
Acquired	Acute idiopathic TTP	
	Secondary TTP	Drugs: oral contraceptive pill, ticlopidine, ciclosporin, mitomycin C Post-bone marrow transplantation Systemic lupus erythematosus Malignancy Pregnancy Infection – HIV, *Escherichia coli* 0157:H7
	Intermittent TTP	Recurrent episodes at unpredictable intervals

HIV, human immunodeficiency virus.

nous heparin is generally contraindicated. The clinical circumstances in DIC can alter very rapidly, and so frequent and serial laboratory monitoring is key to the management.

Thrombotic thrombocytopenic purpura

Thrombotic thrombocytopenic purpura (TTP) is a clinical diagnosis characterized by the classic pentad of features, namely thrombocytopenia (Fig. 14.6), microangiopathic haemolytic anaemia, fluctuating neurological signs, renal impairment and fever. However, up to 35% of patients do not have neurological symptoms or signs at presentation, and the diagnosis of TTP should be suspected in any patient presenting with a microangiopathic haemolytic anaemia and thrombocytopenia in the absence of any other identifiable cause (Table 14.6).

The syndrome is characterized by the formation of platelet microvascular thrombi, which primarily affect the renal and cerebral circulations. The principal abnormality is a deficiency in a protease called ADAMTS13, the function of which is to cleave ultra-large von Willebrand factor (ULVWF) multimers. In the absence of this protease, ULVWF multimers persist in the plasma and result in spontaneous platelet aggregation in the microcirculation. Congenital, idiopathic and secondary forms of TTP exist.

Historically, in the absence of treatment, the mortality rate of TTP was > 90%; however, this has fallen to 10–30% following the institution of urgent plasma exchange for acute TTP. This process

both removes the ULVWF multimers from the patient's circulation and replaces the ADAMTS13 protease in the fresh frozen plasma that is used as replacement fluid. Before commencing plasma exchange, a vascular catheter will need to be inserted, but platelet transfusions should be avoided, even in cases with a severe thrombocytopenia, because these patients rarely bleed, and the addition of allogeneic platelets can lead to further platelet aggregation and worsen the underlying condition. Plasma exchange should be continued daily until at least 2 days after the platelet count normalizes. If plasma exchange is unavailable, infusions of fresh frozen plasma can be given; however, these are associated with an inferior outcome compared with plasma exchange. Immunosuppression may be required in the longer term in idiopathic TTP to prevent relapse of the condition.

Infection in patients with impaired immunity

Patients with a variety of haematological diseases are immunocompromised as a result both of their underlying disease and the treatment required for the condition. Impaired immunity to infection may be the result of neutropenia, lymphocytopenia, hypogammaglobulinaemia or a combination of these abnormalities (Table 14.7).

A number of haematology patients will be severely neutropenic following either inpatient or outpatient aggressive chemotherapy

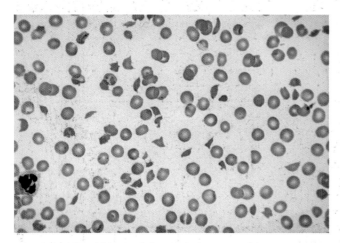

Figure 14.6 Red cell fragments (irregularly shaped cells amongst the normal round red cells) seen on the blood film of a patient with thrombotic thrombocytopenic purpura. Note also the marked thrombocytopenia seen in this blood film.

Table 14.7 Risks of infection in patients with no spleen or hypofunctioning spleen

Incidence	Organisms
Commonly with encapsulated organisms	*Streptococcus pneumoniae* (60%), *Haemophilus influenzae* type b, *Neisseria meningitidis*
Less commonly	*Escherichia coli*, malaria, babesiosis, *Capnocytophaga canimorsus*

regimens or as a result of their underlying disease. It is essential that these patients are counselled and supplied with contact numbers and that they understand the urgent need for hospital admission if they become unwell and/or develop a fever. Many of these patients have indwelling tunnelled intravenous catheters, and line-related infections with Gram-positive organisms are common. On admission, all neutropenic patients with a fever (Fig. 14.7) or other features of infection should be treated promptly with broad spectrum antibiotics according to the local hospital protocols, which will reflect both the spectrum of causative organisms and their local sensitivities. Removal of the tunnelled catheter may be necessary for severe or persistent line-associated infections.

Patients with chronic lymphocytic leukaemia (CLL) often have recurrent infection in the absence of neutropenia, due to the hypogammaglobulinaemia seen in this disorder. Frequent courses of antibiotics may be required, but intravenous immunoglobulins are rarely used, owing to the limited evidence of their efficacy. Recurrent and severe herpes zoster infections may also occur, and prompt treatment with aciclovir should be given at the first suspicion of herpetic lesions developing. Treatment of CLL may involve purine analogues, such as fludarabine, or the monoclonal antibody alemtuzumab (CamPath®; Genzyme). These both impair T-cell function, rendering the patient at risk of *Pneumocystis carinii* pneumonia (PCP) infection or cytomegalovirus (CMV) reactivation. PCP prophylaxis with cotrimoxazole is initiated coincidentally with treatment with these drugs, and polymerase chain reaction monitoring for CMV should be used.

Patients with either functional or anatomical asplenia are at an increased risk of infection with encapsulated organisms, notably *Streptococcus pneumoniae*. It is now recommended that all such patients should be vaccinated against *S. pneumoniae*, *Haemophilus influenzae* and meningococcus, and remain on lifelong prophylactic antibiotics, for example penicillin V (Box 14.5). Counselling regarding the need for prompt treatment with antibiotics in the event of a fever

> **Box 14.5 Recommendations for patients with no spleen or hypofunctioning spleen**
>
> The following vaccinations should be given, ideally, 2 weeks before but alternatively as soon as possible after splenectomy
> - Pneumococcal vaccine (Pneumovax II) (reimmunize every 5 years)
> - *Haemophilus influenzae* type b (Hib) vaccine
> - Meningococcal polysaccharide vaccine for *Neisseria meningitidis* types A and C
>
> All patients should receive lifelong prophylaxis with penicillin V (250 mg twice daily) or erythromycin if penicillin allergic

is important, and patients should be supplied with an information alert card.

Further reading

Allford SL, Hunt BJ, Rose P *et al*. Guidelines on the diagnosis and management of the thrombotic microangiopathic anaemias. *British Journal of Haematology* 2003; **120**: 556–73.

British Committee for Standards in Haematology, Blood Transfusion Task Force. Guidelines for the use of platelet transfusions. *British Journal of Haematology* 2003; **122**: 10–23.

Davies JM, Barnes R, Milligan D *et al*. Update of guidelines for the prevention and treatment of infection in patients with an absent or dysfunctional spleen. *Clinical Medicine* 2002; **2**: 440–3.

Kyle RA, Disperienzi A. Neurological aspects of monoclonal gammopathy of undetermined significance, multiple myeloma, and related disorders. In: Gahrton G, Durie BGM & Samson D, eds. *Multiple Myeloma and Related Disorders*. Arnold, London.

Oscier D, Fegan C, Hillmen P *et al*. Guidelines on the diagnosis and management of chronic lymphocytic leukaemia. *British Journal of Haematology* 2004; **125**: 294–317.

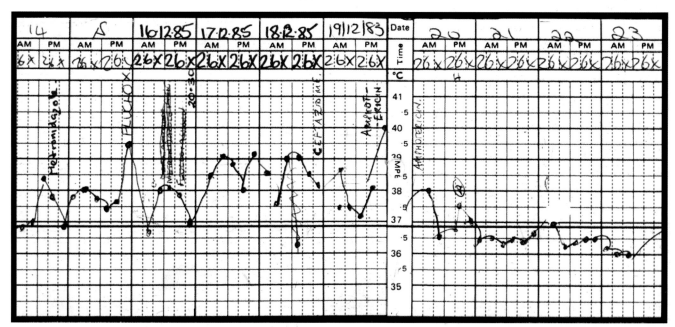

Figure 14.7 Temperature chart showing marked swinging pyrexia in a patient with chronic lymphocytic leukaemia. Fevers of this type are also seen in other immunocompromised patients, such as those with neutropenia.

O'Shaughnessy DF, Atterbury C, Bolton Maggs P *et al*. Guidelines for the use of fresh frozen plasma and cryoprecipitate and cryosupernatant. *British Journal of Haematology* 2004; **126:** 11–28.

Powles R, Sirochi B, Kulkarni S. Investigation and management of hyperleukocytosis in adults. Chapter 3. In: Pinketon R, Rohatiner A & Miles A, eds. *The Effective Prevention and Management of Common Complications of Induction Chemotherapy in Haematological Malignancy*. Aesculapius Medical Press, London, 2003: 33–50.

Rees DC, Olujohungbe AD, Parker NE *et al*. Guidelines for the management of the acute painful crisis in sickle cell disease. *British Journal of Haematology* 2003; **120:** 744–52.

Reinhart WH, Lutolf O, Nydegger U, *et al*. Plasmapheresis for hyperviscosity syndrome in macroglobulinaemia Waldenstrom and multiple myeloma; influence on blood rheology and the microcirculation. *Journal of Laboratory and Clinical Medicine* 1992; **119:** 69–76.

Acknowledgements

The radiographs in Fig. 14.3 were kindly supplied by Dr Alison Page, Consultant Radiologist at the Queen Elizabeth Hospital, Birmingham.

CHAPTER 15

The Future of Haematology: the Impact of Molecular Biology and Gene Therapy

Bella R Patel, Adele K Fielding

OVERVIEW

- The techniques of molecular biology, once confined to research laboratories, are increasingly used in diagnosis and monitoring of a wide variety of haematological disorders and will become standard practice

- Antibodies have found a firm clinical role in the treatment of both malignant and non-malignant haemtological disorders. Other "biological "therapies such as anti-cancer vaccines and viral vectors for gene therapy are entering clinical study and are likely to follow suit

- "Targeted" drug therapies based on known molecular aberrations will play an increasing role

This chapter assesses the impact of advances in science and technology on the practice of haematology and attempts to predict how haematology might change further over the next 10–15 years (Box 15.1).

The major advances in scientific thought and technological development that have already changed the practice of modern haematology are likely to affect both laboratory diagnosis and treatment in the future. The first draft of the sequence of the human genome has now been published and 'genomics' has mushroomed.

Box 15.1 The future of haematology: diagnosis and treatment

Diagnosis
- Increasing automation giving quicker and more reliable results, e.g. automated cross-matching; automated diagnostic polymerase chain reaction
- More DNA/RNA-based diagnosis, allowing increased diagnostic precision, e.g. precise definition of genetic abnormalities
- More 'near patient' testing, allowing rapid screening, e.g. haemoglobinometers, monitoring of anticoagulant treatment

Treatment
- New drugs, e.g. tailored to molecular abnormalities
- New biological agents, e.g. viruses and viral vectors, monoclonal antibodies
- Transplantation across tissue barriers, e.g. cord blood transplantation
- Gene therapy: potential for many haematological disorders

The first clinical study in which gene therapy provided clear clinical benefit to patients has been reported. Another very exciting development that will ultimately affect the practice of haematology is the discovery of the plasticity of postnatal stem cells. The identification of postnatal progenitors that can, *ex vivo*, be expanded and differentiated into many different cell types, ultimately may pave the way for the treatment of solid organ tissue damage as well as correcting genetic disorders of many kinds. Haemopoietic stem cells are the best characterized postnatal stem cells. They are obtained relatively easily, making them an attractive strategy for clinical application. Although the debate about the ethical implications of the use of embryonic stem cells continues in many countries, postnatal stem cells offer a realistic and non-controversial alternative.

The chapter begins with an introduction to genomics and gene therapy, both of which are likely to have a role in most areas of haematological practice in the future. Three specific areas of haematology – haemoglobinopathy, haemophilia, and haematological malignancy – are then examined, in each of which important innovations could be expected to change clinical practice.

Both diagnostically and therapeutically, the identification of the molecular pathology of the underlying disorder will continue to steer the future. The ability to make more accurate diagnoses in haematology is only just beginning to result in improved treatments. Careful clinical studies with well designed correlative science that aims to ask and answer specific questions should remain the basis on which novel developments make their impact on routine practice.

Gene therapy

The term gene therapy is applied to any manoeuvre in which genes or genetically modified cells are introduced into a patient for therapeutic benefit. Successful gene therapy depends on the availability of reliable methods for delivering a gene into selected target cells and subsequently ensuring the regulation of gene expression. Haematological cells are readily accessible for manipulation and so can be genetically modified outside the body and reinfused (Fig. 15.1). The aim in the future perhaps might be to modify the target cells without first removing them from the patient.

Genes that are to be delivered to cells must first be inserted into plasmids. These small circular molecules of double-stranded DNA

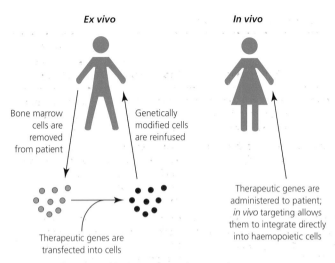

Figure 15.1 *Ex vivo* and *in vivo* gene transfer strategies.

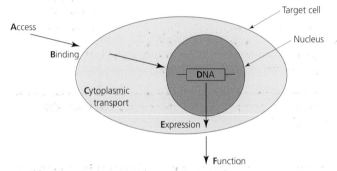

Figure 15.2 ABC of gene therapy. A vector must be able to access the cells to be transduced and bind and penetrate the membrane of the target cell. Once inside the nucleus, the exogenous DNA must be integrated into the cellular genome if stable expression is required. Gene expression must be at a high enough level and sufficiently regulated for clinical benefit. For gene therapy applications, where it is crucial to achieve gene expression in the progeny of the target (modified) cells, it is important to use a vector that stably inserts its genes into the chromosome of the host cell, and retrovirus vectors are the most suitable for this purpose. For direct *in vivo* gene delivery, vector attachment to a specific target cell is a vital additional requirement. Such vector targeting is at last beginning to look like a realistic possibility.

derived from bacteria can then be used to transfer therapeutic genes to cells using DNA delivery vehicles known as vectors (Fig. 15.2). Vectors are either viral or non-viral based. The former have evolved natural mechanisms to deliver genomes into cells, making them ideal vehicles for use in gene therapy. Considerable work in developing viral and non-viral vector systems is underway to try to achieve the steps outlined above. The ultimate choice depends upon the experimental or clinical setting (Table 15.1).

To date, most successful gene therapy applications have employed retroviral vectors (Table 15.2), primarily because of their ability to stably insert into the chromosome of the host cell. This is crucial for achieving adequate gene expression in the progeny of the target cells.

The most successful application of this approach is in patients with X-linked severe combined immunodeficiency syndrome (SCID). The syndrome results from a mutation in the gene encoding the interleukin-2 (IL-2) receptor γ chain (IL2RG), as a result of which patients do not make T and natural killer (NK) cells, and have impaired B-cell function. Correction of the genetic defect involves exposing autologous bone marrow cells to high titre retroviral vector bearing the correct *IL2RG* gene. The transduced haemopoietic cells are then reinfused into the patients. Significant immune reconstitution was seen in the majority of patients treated with this approach – a major success. However, three cases of T-cell leukaemia in children treated by this method were reported. In two of the three cases, leukaemic expansions were from gene-corrected T-cell clones, due to integration of the vector close to the *LMO2* gene promoter, resulting in aberrant expression of the LMO2 transcription factor, a phenomenon known as insertional mutagenesis. What remains unclear for future studies is to what extent retroviral vectors *per se* are responsible for mutagenic events. Particular risks in these patients that contributed to the insertional mutagenesis included the high transduction rate of the vector, the young age of the patients and the strong selective advantage given to transduced cells by the correction of the genetic defect. Intense efforts to elucidate the exact mechanism of these events continues. Despite these problems, the great potential for gene transfer technologies to treat and cure genetic diseases continues to spur interest in this field.

Table 15.1 Gene therapy strategies

Strategy	Potential application
Corrective replacement	Sickle cell disease: to replace the point mutation that causes the substitution of valine for glutamine on the sixth amino acid residue of the β globin chain
Corrective gene addition	Haemophilia: to introduce a gene for missing coagulation protein
Corrective antisense	Low grade non-Hodgkin's lymphoma (NHL) treatment: to introduce antisense oligonucleotides, preventing Bcl-2 overexpression, which is responsible for the failure of the lymphoma cells to undergo apoptosis
Pharmacological	Continuous production of interferon α, erythropoietin, or other therapeutic proteins
Cytotoxic	Leukaemia: targeted delivery of cytotoxic proteins
Prophylactic	Chemoprotection: drug resistance genes introduced into haemopoietic stem cells, conferring resistant phenotype, thus protecting against chemotherapeutic agents
Immunostimulatory	Idiotypic vaccination: in B-cell tumours, such as NHL and myeloma, the variable region sequences of the surface immunoglobulin of the tumour cell provide a tumour-specific antigen against which an individualized vaccine for each patient can be produced
Replicating virus therapy	Oncolytic viruses may be used to directly kill transformed cells

Table 15.2 Viral vector systems for gene delivery in haematology

Vector system	Advantages	Disadvantages	Potential uses	Examples of clinical trials in haematology
Adenovirus	Short-term expression	Transduces haemopoietic cells poorly; short-term expression only	Where only short-term expression is needed	Haemophilia (safe, but ineffective in this context)
AAV	Long-term expression is possible	Transduces haemopoietic cells poorly	Transduces muscle and liver cells well; this feature can be used to express proteins	Ongoing in haemophilia (factor IX deficiency)
Oncoretrovirus	Integrates, long-term expression possible, transduces haemopoietic cells well, including stem cells	Only transduces cycling cells; risk of insertional mutagenesis	Long-term modification of stem cells and their progeny. Modification of T cells	Gene transfer of suicide genes to T cells following allogeneic BMT. Stem cell transduction for correction of X-linked SCID
Lentivirus	Integrates, long-term expression possible, transduces haemopoietic cells well, including stem cells	Many lentiviral vectors are derived from HIV, causing theoretical safety concerns	Long-term modification of stem cells and their progeny	Currently only for HIV

AAV, adeno-associated virus; BMT, bone marrow transplant; HIV, human immunodeficiency virus; SCID, severe combined immunodeficiency syndrome.

Genomics and proteomics

Genomics can be defined as 'the systematic study of all the genes of an organism'. Recently, the number of genes in the human genome has been estimated at being between 30 000 and 40 000, many less than previously thought. The function of most of these genes currently remains unknown, although it is likely that this will not always be the case. It is now possible to obtain a profile of which genes are expressed in a given cell or tissue under defined conditions by means of cDNA arrays, which are thousands of unique DNA probes robotically deposited onto a solid matrix or 'DNA chip' (Fig. 15.3). To profile gene expression in the tissue of interest, messenger RNA (mRNA) is isolated, copied into DNA labelled with a fluorescent dye and then used to probe the DNA chip to obtain an expression profile. A huge amount of data can be gathered in this manner, but to turn this into interpretable information requires considerable computing capacity. The processing and interpretation of the data obtained is known as bioinformatics. The best characterized clinical application of gene profiling is in patients with diffuse large B-cell and follicular lymphomas. In recent years, several large scale studies involving microarray-based gene expression profiling have identified novel prognostic subgroups within each of these lymphoma types. Studies of gene expression can therefore provide a molecular predictor of survival that may be used to inform treatment. In addition, such profiles elucidate the underlying biology of diseases as well as yielding information about the function of unidentified genes. For example, in patients with follicular lymphoma, gene signatures that predict length of survival were found to belong to cells of the immune system. This finding illustrates the importance of immune responses in determining the fate of patients with malignant disorders.

There is emerging evidence for a new mechanism of post-transcriptional regulation of gene expression by micro RNAs. These small non-coding RNAs are thought to target mRNA for degradation, thereby affecting post-transcriptional gene expression. Micro RNA gene expression profiles have recently been demonstrated to predict prognosis in chronic lymphocytic leukaemia (CLL). The future is likely to see further characterization of these molecules in the diagnoses and treatment of leukaemias (Fig. 15.4).

Proteomics, the systematic study of all the proteins in a cell, tissue or organ, may ultimately be more useful than genomics. However, the technical hurdles are much greater, not least because of the vast number and complexity of the proteins to be studied. Improved methods for gel separation of proteins and improved image analysis are likely to make study of the proteome a legitimate goal.

Haemoglobinopathies

The identification of the precise mutations associated with many forms of hereditary anaemias will allow routine characterization by nucleic acid sequence analysis, facilitating the use of disease-specific diagnostic tests based on polymerase chain reaction. This will provide more precise prognostic information for affected individuals as well as accurate identification of affected embryos. As reliable prenatal diagnosis at an early stage will be available, so will an increasing range of prenatal treatment options.

For patients affected by hereditary anaemias, such as sickle cell disease and thalassaemia, advances in transplantation immunol-

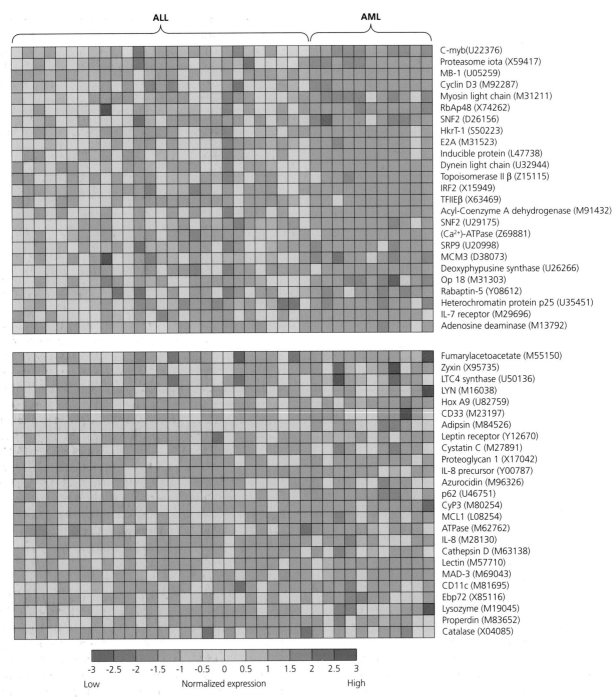

Figure 15.3 Microarray technology allows the analysis of thousands of different genes simultaneously. Reproduced from Aitman TJ (*British Medical Journal* 2001; **323**: 611–5) and adapted from Golub TR *et al.* (*Science* 1999; **286**: 531–7).

ogy are likely to permit transplantation across tissue barriers with reduced immunosuppression, making bone marrow transplantation a treatment option for more affected patients. In addition, gene therapy for these disorders could provide another potentially curative strategy, although the genetic correction of hereditary anaemias still presents complex challenges. In sickle cell disease, for example, delivery of normal copies of the β globin gene to haemopoietic stem cells will be insufficient for cure. As continued Hb S production would be damaging, the mutated β globin genes must also be removed.

Most recently, a relevant potential new gene correction strategy has been described. This strategy uses DNA cleaving enzymes to induce a double-stranded break into DNA at specific sites near mutations. Subsequently, a natural cell repair mechanism, known as homologous recombination, repairs the damage by using a wild type (unmutated) sequence as a template. The end result is correction of the mutant sequence. The advantages of this approach are avoidance of insertional mutagenesis and no requirement for long-term expression of either the DNA cleaving enzymes or the normal template.

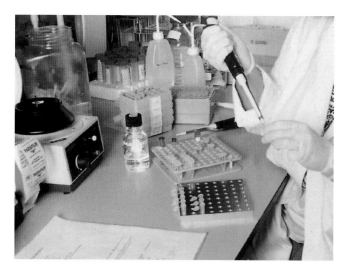

Figure 15.4 Gene therapy may provide a curative strategy for a variety of disorders, including haemoglobinopathies, coagulation disorders, and other single gene disorders.

As our understanding of the molecular events that contribute to gene control develops, so does the opportunity of developing novel therapies. In the case of sickle cell disease, pharmacological manipulation of the fetal haemoglobin (Hb F) gene is being used to ameliorate the disease phenotype. Classes of drugs used for this purpose include hypomethylating agents and inhibitors of histone deacetylases, both of which raise Hb F levels by increasing the expression of γ globin genes.

Haemophilia

The modern diagnosis of haemophilia relies on identifying specific characteristic mutations within the factor VIII or IX genes. This approach facilitates accurate carrier diagnosis as well as identification of affected embryos. Mutational analysis is also extremely informative in predicting the severity of disease and likelihood of inhibitor formation, which may alter disease management.

The emergence of gene replacement therapy in haemophilia was built on the success of recombinant coagulation proteins following the identification and cloning of both the factor VIII and IX genes. These treatments are now used in preference to plasma derivatives, which obviates problems with transmissible infections. Undoubtedly, recombinant technology and the production of recombinant coagulation factors have significantly improved the prospects for all patients with bleeding diathesis and those who have developed the serious complication of inhibitor formation (Fig. 15.5). The future

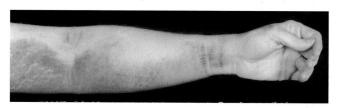

Figure 15.5 Haemophilic patient with inhibitors and severe spontaneous bleeding. Currently, the development of inhibitors represents one of the biggest problems facing patients with haemophilia.

is likely to see a more complete repertoire of recombinant clotting products used to treat people with genetic bleeding disorders.

Because haemophilia results from a single gene defect in which protein levels need only be increased minimally to give significant clinical benefit, it is a condition that is, in theory, extremely amenable to a gene therapy approach. A number of phase I trials reported the potential for such an approach. Subsequently, five successor trials in the 1990s, each using different gene delivery systems, were conducted. They reported initial factor level increases in some individuals but these were not sustained. Considerable work on the development of new vectors for haemophilia gene therapy suggests that cure of haemophilia by gene therapy remains a very realistic possibility.

Haematological malignancy

An understanding of the molecular mechanism of malignant transformation in malignant disorders forms the basis for improved diagnostic sensitivity and the monitoring of minimal residual disease. This paves the way for more directed treatment interventions, including the eventual possibility of targeting the causative genetic defects. The new genetic information available from genomic studies will increasingly be used to classify malignancies and may provide novel therapeutic targets. A recent example of a molecular discovery that will lead to improved diagnostic precision is the finding of acquired recurrent activating mutations in the Janus kinase 2 (*JAK2*) gene in myeloproliferative disorders (MPD). By far the vast majority (65–97%) of these mutations are found in patients with polycythaemia rubra vera, less often in essential thrombocythaemia (32–57%) and idiopathic myelofibrosis (43–50%). These findings are likely to lead to a revision in the diagnostic criteria of MPD and may, in the future, serve as a potential target for drug therapy.

Future therapies for haematological malignancies
Novel pharmaceutical approaches
Tyrosine kinase inhibitors
The success of imatinib, an Abl-specific tyrosine kinase inhibitor used to treat patients with chronic myeloid leukaemia, has demonstrated the potential of therapies targeted at molecular abnormalities (Fig. 15.6). Further examples of how an understanding of molecular mechanisms of mutagenesis is helping to generate novel therapies are ongoing trials of FLT3 inhibitors in patients with acute myeloid leukaemia (AML). Their use is based upon recent characterization of the FLT3 tyrosine kinase receptor mutations (internal tandem duplications and point mutations in the activating loop of the kinase domain) found in approximately one-third of patients with AML. These mutations result in constitutive FLT3 tyrosine kinase activity with consequent dysregulation of cell proliferation and apoptosis, which are associated with a poor prognosis.

Monoclonal antibodies
The remarkable success of anti-CD20 has paved the way for further therapeutic success with antibody therapies. Their unique mechanisms of action, lack of cross-resistance and non-additive toxicities make them attractive anticancer therapies. In most cases, these therapies are likely to be used in conjunction with more established

(a)

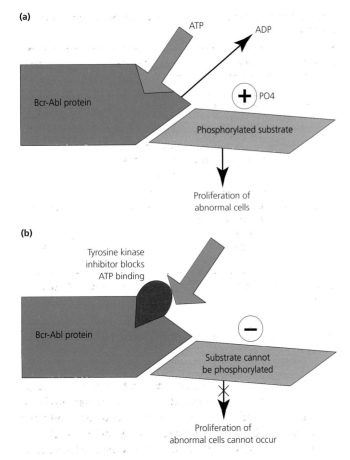

Figure 15.6 (a) Aberrant protein Bcr–Abl is produced in chronic myeloid leukaemia (CML) cells as a result of translocation of material from chromosome 9 to chromosome 22. It binds adenosine triphosphate (ATP), then transfers phosphate groups to tyrosine residues on various substrate proteins. Downstream events lead to proliferation of the CML cells. (b) When imatinib binds to the ATP binding site of Bcr–Abl, the tyrosine kinase activity of this protein is inhibited and the events leading to proliferation of the CML cells cannot occur.

chemotherapy regimens rather than as a single agent. Substantial study will be required to determine the best way to integrate their activity into standard chemotherapy regimens (Box 15.2).

Angiogenesis inhibitors

Angiogenesis has been shown to play a critical role in tumorigenesis and susceptibility to intensive chemotherapy. Vascular growth is mediated by the local proliferation and migration of vessel wall-associated endothelial cells in response to growth factors, such as vascular endothelial growth factor (VEGF) via its tyrosine kinase receptor; these are therefore attractive targets for therapy. Pathological angiogenesis is well characterized in multiple myeloma, where multiple myeloma cells directly produce VEGF and induce VEGF secretion by bone marrow stromal cells. AML blasts have also been shown to constitutively express proangiogenic factors as a result of interactions with neighbouring non-leukaemic cells. Several antiangiogenic molecules are now in clinical trial and, as the complex biology of angiogenesis unfolds, it is likely that further therapeutic targets will be developed.

Modulators of gene expression

Deregulated control of genes by aberrant transcription factors appears to be critical for tumour development. In AML, chromosomal translocations yield abnormal transcription factors that, in turn, either activate genes critical for cell growth or repress genes important for normal cellular differentiation. These aberrant transcription factors modulate gene regulation by recruiting histone deacetylases (HDACs), and thus HDACs are a compelling therapeutic target for therapy. Mutations in *ras* oncogenes have been identified in approximately 25% of AML patients. These mutations lead to constitutive Ras activation. Farnesyl transferase inhibitors interfere with the activation of Ras, making them attractive targets for drug therapy.

Modulators of apoptosis

Apoptosis is an intrinsic cell death programme that is regulated by the balance of proapoptotic and antiapoptotic proteins. Imbalances of these regulatory proteins can endow cells with a selective survival advantage that promotes malignancy. Emerging knowledge about the molecular mechanisms involved in apoptosis and how they are dysregulated in cancer heralds new drug targets.

Overexpression of antiapoptotic Bcl-2 proteins, characteristic of follicular lymphoma, can be targeted using antisense oligodeoxynucleotides directed towards Bcl-2 mRNA, or by directly attacking the proteins themselves with small molecule drugs. Such drugs are currently undergoing clinical evaluation, with phase III trials underway or recently completed for relapsed or refractory CLL, AML and myeloma.

Other therapies

Drug therapies that indirectly modulate tumour necrosis factor (TNF) activity are also being developed. The nuclear factor kappa B (NF-κB) family of transcription factors is known to inhibit TNF-induced apoptosis by affecting the activity of several antiapoptotic genes. NF-κB is inhibited by the IκB proteins. Current strategies that modulate TNF activity do so by increasing the activity of these inhibitory proteins, thereby reducing NF-κB inhibition of TNF. This is achieved by interfering with the degradation of IκB proteins by the proteasome. Proteasome inhibitors in clinical use include bortezomib (PS-341 – Velcade®; Ortho Biotech), which has recently been approved for treatment of refractory myeloma and is in clinical testing for several types of lymphoma in which abnormal elevations in NF-κB activity have been demonstrated. It is likely that proteasome inhibitors affect several other regulatory proteins involved in apoptosis. Elucidation of these pathways will expand the number of available apoptosis-based therapies.

Immunotherapy in haematological malignancy

The activity of the immune system in eliminating haematological malignancy has been exploited for many years by the use of allogeneic bone marrow transplant. The toxicity of this approach and its limited applicability to older individuals have led to a more subtle approach using reduced intensity conditioning. Here, the action of donor T cells either in the graft or donor lymphocyte infusion following transplant, rather than dose intensification, promotes engraftment and tumour eradication and generates a graft-versus-leukaemia (GVL) effect. Considerable ongoing work will focus on developing truly minimally toxic regimens that rely exclusively on GVL for tumour control. Such an approach, if successful, would become a feasible treatment option for elderly or infirm patients as well as an acceptable strategy for allogeneic transplantation in patients with indolent malignancies (Table 15.3).

The long-term risk of graft-versus-host disease (GVHD), also mediated by donor T cells, has led to the search for alternative immunological pathways that confer a more targeted GVL effect. One such strategy employs natural killer (NK) cells. Experimental evidence suggests that these cells predominantly attack the malignant haemopoietic cells of the host but not other tissues that are common targets for T-cell-mediated GVHD. Other strategies aimed at enhancing the

Table 15.3 Immunotherapeutic approaches to the therapy of haematological malignancy

Approach	Rationale	Advantages	Disadvantages
Conventional (high-dose) allogeneic transplantation	Marrow ablative conditioning overcomes host rejection whilst eradicating underlying disease	Extremely effective for rapidly progressive disease such as acute leukaemia and high grade lymphoma	Highly toxic procedure
RIC transplantation	GVL effects are exploited while immunosuppression overcomes host rejection	Conditioning regimen is less toxic	Late GVHD. GVL effects not sufficient or rapid enough to control rapidly progressive disease

GVHD, graft-versus-host disease; GVL, graft-versus-leukaemia; RIC, reduced intensity conditioning.

immune response to malignant cells, such as, for example, idiotypic vaccination in lymphoma, are likely to play an important role, particularly in the setting of minimal residual disease and following reduced intensity conditioned transplantation. A variety of vaccine approaches for multiple myeloma and lymphomas are currently being tested in clinical trials (Table 15.4). Approaches to immunotherapy in haematological malignancies are summarized in Table 15.5.

Novel therapies must be developed in the context of exisiting treatment. Although novel therapies are usually tested in the late stages of malignant disease, this is unlikely to be the optimal time for patients to benefit from such therapies so that disappointing results from early stage clinical studies should be interpreted wtih caution.

Enhancement of the safety of exisiting treatments and increasing the number of people to whom exisiting treatments are applicable

---

Box 15.2 **The future of antibody therapy for lymphoma?**

Radioimmunotherapy
- The use of monoclonal antibodies to deliver radioisotopes has shown great efficacy in the treatment of lymphoma
- Targeted radiotherapy using the pan-leucocyte antigen CD45 is being studied for myeloablation before stem cell transplantation

Antibody delivery of immunotoxins
- Drugs or toxins can be conjugated to antibodies to increase potency
- Target antigens that are internalized are needed for this approach

Novel target antigens
- Target antigens, other than CD20 for which this approach is being developed clinically, include CD22, HLA-DR, CD52, anti-CD80 therapy for B-cell lymphoma, and anti-CD3

Targeted delivery of oncolytic viruses via viral display of single chain antibodies
- *In vitro* studies and work in animal models suggest that this may be a feasible approach

---

Table 15.4 New treatment and prevention strategies

Strategy	Rationale	Advantages	Disadvantages
Vaccination			
Antigen-specific vaccines	Tumour antigens invoke a host-specific immune response towards malignant cells bearing these antigens, resulting in eradication of the cells. Clinical trials ongoing	Such an approach provides greater control in targeting the antitumour response	Tumour antigens can change over time (antigen drift), rendering the vaccine ineffective
Peptide vaccines	Amino acid motifs recognized by recipient T cells form effective immunogens	Invokes a more targeted and specific immune response	Limited to patients expressing the specific HLA molecules
Cell based-vaccines	The tumour cell (with a broad spectrum of tumour antigens) is used as an antigen source	Increases efficacy and specificity of immune response	Technically demanding as requires whole tumour cell isolation and characterization
Dendritic cell vaccine	DCs are potent antigen presenting cells	DCs are capable of priming effective T cell responses against tumour-specific antigens	The inability to direct antigen loaded DCs to lymphoid organs, for presentation to T cells
Adoptive T-cell therapy	Here T cells isolated from the patient or other individuals are modified or expanded *ex vivo* before transfer back to the patient	Overcomes the immune suppression of the host and subsequent inability to generate an adequate antitumour response	Requires sufficient numbers of T cells to exert a measurable anti-tumour effect. There are inherent problems with expanding T cells *ex vivo* and sustaining numbers upon infusion. Risk of GVHD

DCs, dendritic cells; GVHD, graft-versus-host disease; HLA, human leucocyte antigen.

Table 15.5 Scientific techniques and approaches that have made major contributions to modern haematology

Technique	Applications in haematology
Gene cloning and sequencing allow identification, characterization, and manipulation of genes responsible for specific products or diseases	Elucidation of the molecular pathology of disease and diagnostic tests based on the polymerase chain reaction
Polymerase chain reaction is a highly sensitive and versatile technique for amplifying very small quantities of DNA. Amplification of RNA molecules is possible after initial reverse transcription of RNA into DNA (RT-PCR)	Rapid diagnosis of infectious diseases in immunocompromised patients (for example, hepatitis C); minimal residual disease detection in haematological malignancies where the molecular defect is known; carrier detection and antenatal diagnosis in haemophilias and hereditary anaemias
Monoclonal antibodies allow immunohistochemistry of tissue and cells, analysis and cell sorting with fluorescence activated cell sorter, and cell purification	Increased diagnostic precision, 'positive purging', *ex vivo* gene delivery, and *ex vivo* expansion of progenitor cells are possible as a result of the fact that populations of haemopoietic cells containing a high proportion of primitive progenitors can be isolated
Mammalian tissue culture and gene transfer to mammalian cells provide methods for studying gene expression. Reporter genes can be used to study gene expression in cell lines *in vitro*. Transgenic animals can be created by inserting intact or manipulated genes into the germ line of an animal, providing an *in vivo* model of gene function	Allows gene therapy, tissue engineering, and study of gene expression and function
Protein engineering and construction of recombinant proteins allow production of large quantities of human proteins. Proteins with modified or novel functions can be rationally designed and produced	Recombinant drugs (for example, the haemopoietic growth factors), antibody engineering to produce therapeutic antibodies, recombinant blood products free from risk of viral contamination
Small interfering RNA (siRNA) technology is a new approach for blocking the production of a protein by specific degradation of the messenger RNA that encodes the protein	The high potency of siRNA and the relative ease of application have led to broad implementation of the method in many aspects of life science research. The combination of developments in its application and in siRNA libraries to cover whole genomes has further enabled genome-wide, high-throughput functional screening

RT-PCR, reverse transcriptase polymerase chain reaction.

will remain an important aspect of the treatment of haematological malignancy. "Pharmacogenomics" may offer us the opportunity to identify the genetic mechanims affecting the responses to and toxicity of chemotherapy in individual patients and offer the opportunity to modify doses or combinations on an individual basis.

Further reading

Dave SS, Wright G. Prediction of survival in follicular lymphoma based on molecular features of tumor-infiltrating immune cells. *New England Journal of Medicine* 2004; **351:** 2159–69.

Emilien G, Ponchon M, Caldas C *et al.* Impact of genomics on drug discovery and clinical medicine. *Quarterly Journal of Medicine* 2000; **93:** 391–423.

Frohling S, Scholl C, Gilliland DG *et al.* Genetics of myeloid malignancies: pathogenetic and clinical implications. *Journal of Clinical Oncology* 2005; **23:** 6285–95.

Ilidge TM, Bayne MC. Antibody therapy of lymphoma. *Expert Opinion in Pharmacotherapy* 2001; 2: 953–61.

Mannucci PM, Tuddenham EG. The hemophilias – from royal genes to gene therapy. *New England Journal of Medicine* 2001; **344:** 1773–9.

Mauro MJ, O'Dwyer M, Heinrich MC *et al.* STI571: a paradigm of new agents for cancer therapeutics. *Journal of Clinical Oncology* 2002; **20:** 325–34.

Miller DG, Stamatoyannopoulos G. Gene therapy for hemophilia. *New England Journal of Medicine* 2001; **344:** 1782–4.

Roth DA, Tawa NE Jr, O'Brien JM *et al.* Nonviral transfer of the gene encoding coagulation factor VIII in patients with severe hemophilia A. *New England Journal of Medicine* 2001; **344:** 1735–42.

Seth P. Vector mediated gene cancer therapy. *Cancer Biology and Therapy* 2005; **4:** 512–17.

Shipp MA, Ross KN, Tamayo P *et al.* Diffuse large B-cell lymphoma outcome prediction by gene-expression profiling and supervised machine learning. *Nature Medicine* 2002; **8:** 68–74.

Box 15.3 **Glossary**

General molecular biology
- Histone deacetylases (HDACs): histones are proteins that bind to DNA. HDACs are enzymes that catalyse the removal of acetyl groups from histone proteins, thereby affecting and usually increasing gene transcription
- Oncogene/tumour suppressor gene: a gene that normally directs cell growth. If altered, can promote or allow the uncontrolled growth of cells and malignant transformation
- Polymerase chain reaction: process by which genes or gene segments can be rapidly, conveniently, and accurately copied, producing up to 1012 copies of the original sequence in a few hours
- Recombinant DNA: any DNA sequence that does not occur naturally but is formed by joining DNA segments from different sources
- Reverse transcription: process by which RNA is used as a template for the production of a DNA copy: cDNA
- Transcription factor: protein that is able to bind to chromosomal DNA close to a gene and thereby regulates the expression of the gene

Haematology and immunology
- Adoptive immunotherapy: the transfer of immune cells for therapeutic benefit
- Apoptosis: programmed cell death
- Developmental plasticity: the ability of postnatal stem cells to generate differentiated cells beyond their own tissue boundaries
- Embryonic stem cells: derived from mammalian embryos in the blastocyst stage. They have the ability to self renew, differentiate and generate any terminally differentiated cell in the body
- Genomics: the systematic study of the human genome
- Haemopoietic stem cell: a type of postnatal/adult stem cell that is tissue specific. Can give rise to all lineages of haemopoietic cells
- Immunophenotype: the cell surface markers on any given cell detected by the use of monoclonal antibodies
- Insertional mutagenesis: a mutation is caused by the introduction of foreign DNA sequences into a gene
- Minimal residual disease: cancer that is still present in the body after treatment but remains undetectable by conventional means, e.g. light microscopy
- Proteasome: a barrel-shaped multiprotein complex that can digest other proteins into short polypeptides and amino acids
- Proteomics: the systematic study of the human proteome
- Transgenic animals: animals with an intact or manipulated gene inserted into their germ line

Index